Wills Eye
Strabismus Atlas

Wills Eye Strabismus Atlas

Second Edition

Leonard B Nelson MD
Director, The Wills Eye Strabismus Center
Co-Director, Department of Pediatric Ophthalmology and
Ocular Genetics, Wills Eye Hospital
Associate Professor of Ophthalmology and Pediatrics
Jefferson Medical Center
Thomas Jefferson University
Philadelphia, Pennsylvania, USA

Robert A Catalano MD
Associate Clinical Professor of Ophthalmology
College of Physicians and Surgeons
Columbia University
New York, New York, USA

Foreword

Julia A Haller MD

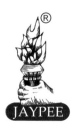

JAYPEE BROTHERS MEDICAL PUBLISHERS (P) LTD
Philadelphia • New Delhi • London • Panama

Jaypee Brothers Medical Publishers (P) Ltd

Headquarters

Jaypee Brothers Medical Publishers (P) Ltd
4838/24, Ansari Road, Daryaganj
New Delhi 110 002, India
Phone: +91-11-43574357
Fax: +91-11-43574314
Email: jaypee@jaypeebrothers.com

Overseas Offices

J.P. Medical Ltd
83, Victoria Street, London
SW1H 0HW (UK)
Phone: +44-2031708910
Fax: +02-03-0086180
Email: info@jpmedpub.com

Jaypee-Highlights.
Medical Publishers Inc
City of Knowledge, Bld. 237
Clayton, Panama City, Panama
Phone: +1 507-301-0496
Fax: +1 507-301-0499
Email: cservice@jphmedical.com

Jaypee Medical Inc.
The Bourse
111 South Independence Mall East
Suite 835, Philadelphia, PA 19106, USA
Phone: +1 267-519-9789
Email: jpmed.us@gmail.com

Jaypee Brothers
Medical Publishers (P) Ltd
17/1-B Babar Road, Block-B
Shaymali, Mohammadpur
Dhaka-1207, Bangladesh
Mobile: +08801912003485
Email: jaypeedhaka@gmail.com

Jaypee Brothers
Medical Publishers (P) Ltd
Shorakhute, Kathmandu
Nepal
Phone: +00977-9841528578
Email: jaypee.nepal@gmail.com

Website: www.jaypeebrothers.com
Website: www.jaypeedigital.com

Inquiries for bulk sales may be solicited at: jaypee@jaypeebrothers.com

Wills Eye Strabismus Atlas

Second Edition: 2014
ISBN 978-93-5152-185-3
Printed at Replika Press Pvt. Ltd.

Foreword

Let your eyes look directly forward, and your gaze be straight before you.
Proverbs 4:25

For all of human history, until quite recently, the biblical injunction mandating a direct, straight gaze was out of reach for many. Remarkable progress in the last decades, however, has dramatically changed that situation. This second edition of the Wills Eye Strabismus Atlas by Nelson and Catalano builds on the latest advances in the fields of ocular motility and sensorimotor innervation: updating and expanding their classic text of 1989, this book serves as a guide for all who aim to diagnose and correct abnormalities of gaze.

This authoritative volume includes not only new research into sensory and motor abnormalities, but the latest advances in the diagnosis of the many strabismus disorders encountered in pediatric ophthalmology. With revised, state-of-the-art diagrams and illustrations in full color, the book is rich in clinical material: expanded with extensive use of cases from the Wills Eye Strabismus Center, directed by Dr Nelson. It serves as a comprehensive, readable, practical guide to strabismologists, ophthalmologists, residents, students, and health care practitioners at every level in the field.

The Proverbial gaze that is straight and direct: this second edition of the *Wills Eye Strabismus Atlas*, replete with essential new diagnostic and management guidelines, is a *sine qua non* for those dedicated to that goal.

Julia A Haller MD
Ophthalmologist-in-Chief
The William Tasman Endowed Chair in Ophthalmology
Wills Eye Hospital
Professor and Chair of Ophthalmology
Thomas Jefferson University
Philadelphia, Pennsylvania, USA

Each year, we observe residents as they anxiously begin their first rotation in pediatric ophthalmology. With little knowledge and experience, these residents embark on a clinical course to obtain the necessary information and data to diagnose disorders of ocular motility and to formulate appropriate treatment plans. It is important for residents not only to be able to detect abnormalities in binocular function but to clearly understand the normal anatomic and physiologic relations in ocular motility. In this atlas, we have provided the reader with important and unique features of ocular anatomy, sensory physiology, and tests of sensory status and ocular alignment. With an understanding of normal binocular function, the reader can better appreciate the specific strabismus disorders and syndromes that are discussed in the second part of the atlas. This second edition of this atlas brings a number of changes to a publication which had been well received among residents, fellows, and the pediatric ophthalmology community in general as an excellent teaching and educational treatise on strabismus. The second edition is titled, *Wills Eye Strabismus Atlas*, as Wills Eye Hospital in Philadelphia, Pennsylvania, USA, is a rich storehouse of clinical material and provided the major background for this book. The Pediatric Ophthalmology and Ocular Genetics Department at Wills Eye Hospital cares for thousands of children and adults with strabismus and provides a rare opportunity for the study of an extremely wide variety of ocular motility disorders. The major change in this atlas is that it is in color which makes for an even better teaching publication. We hope that this second edition will continue to serve as an extremely helpful teaching and review manual for those interested in ocular motility.

Leonard B Nelson MD
Robert A Catalano MD

Acknowledgments

It is with pleasure and gratitude that we acknowledge the many individuals who helped make this publication possible. Laurie Maimone illustrated the first edition of this publication, and we remain very appreciative of her expertise as an artist. We are also indebted to Jack Scully, Roger Barone, and Michael Mehu for their tireless work photographing many patients and making numerous composites. The insight and assistance of Joe Rusko and Marco Ulloa Jr of M/s Jaypee Brothers Medical Publishers have seen this edition to fruition. Finally, we would like to thank all the residents and fellows whom we have had the privilege and opportunity to have taught. Their many questions and concerns for patient care have stimulated us to produce this treatise.

Contents

1

Anatomic Relationships

GROSS ANATOMY OF THE EXTRAOCULAR MUSCLES

The six extraocular muscles have names corresponding to their location and the direction they traverse to insert on the globe (Figs 1.1A to C). Four muscles follow a straight course from the apex of the orbit to the eye and are termed "rectus muscles". Each rectus muscle inserts on the sclera of the eye in a position corresponding to its name, i.e. a superior, inferior, medial and lateral. Two "oblique muscles" also insert on the eye. The superior oblique muscle proceeds forward from the apex of the orbit to become tendinous just before passing through a fibrocartilaginous loop, the "trochlea", attached to the trochlear fossa of the frontal bone. From here the tendon passes under the superior rectus muscle to insert posterior to the equator of the eye in the superolateral quadrant. The inferior oblique muscle arises from the anterior margin of the floor of the orbit, from the orbital surface of the maxilla, lateral to the nasolacrimal groove. It passes posteriorly, laterally and superiorly to insert posterior to the equator of the eye in the inferotemporal quadrant.

The rectus muscles average approximately 37 mm in length, with tendons 3 mm (medial rectus) to 7 mm (lateral rectus) long. The superior oblique muscle is approximately 40 mm in length and its tendon is 20 mm long. The inferior oblique is the shortest of the extraocular muscles, extending only 37 mm with no or a very short tendon of 1–2 mm. The width of the insertions of the rectus muscles averages 9–10 mm. The width of the insertions of the oblique muscles varies considerably, measuring 7–18 mm for the superior oblique and 5–14 mm for the inferior oblique.

The four rectus muscles arise from the apex of the orbit, along with the origins of the superior oblique muscle and the levator palpebrae (Fig. 1.2). The circular arrangement of their insertions around the optic canal and part of the superior orbital fissure is called the "annulus of Zinn". The optic nerve and ophthalmic artery as well as the third and sixth cranial nerves pass through the annulus of Zinn into the cone-shaped space (the "muscle cone") created by the bellies of the rectus muscles.

INNERVATION AND BLOOD SUPPLY TO THE EXTRAOCULAR MUSCLES

Three cranial nerves innervate all the intraocular and extraocular muscles of the eye (Figs 1.3A and B). The brainstem nuclei of these three cranial nerves are shown in Figure 1.3A, from the work of Warwick.

The third cranial nerve (CN III), or the "oculomotor nerve", innervates the majority of the extraocular muscles and all the intraocular muscles of the eye. The nuclear complex of this nerve is located in the periaqueductal gray matter of the mesencephalon at the level of the superior colliculus. A single midline collection of cells innervates both levator palpebrae muscles. This is the only nucleus that bilaterally innervates extraocular muscles. The nucleus to the superior rectus muscle is the only nucleus in the third nerve complex that innervates a contralateral muscle. After leaving the brainstem, the fibers to the levator palpebrae and superior rectus muscles travel together as the "upper division" of the third cranial nerve (CN III$_1$) (Fig. 1.3B). The medial rectus, the inferior rectus and the inferior oblique muscles are innervated by ipsilateral nuclei, and their fibers

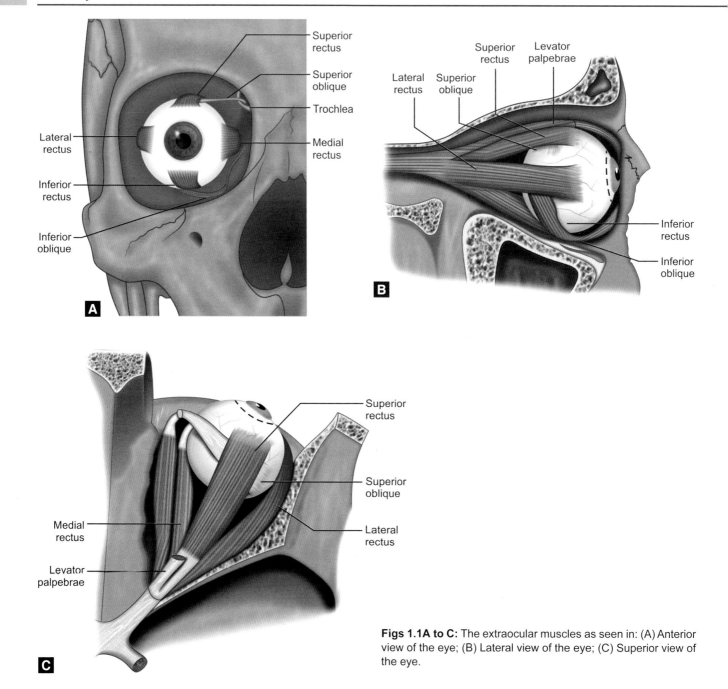

Figs 1.1A to C: The extraocular muscles as seen in: (A) Anterior view of the eye; (B) Lateral view of the eye; (C) Superior view of the eye.

travel together as the lower division (CN III$_2$). The third cranial nerve also supplies parasympathetic innervations to the intraocular muscles of the eye via the "accessory" or "Edinger-Westphal" nucleus. Parasympathetic fibers travel with the nerve to the inferior oblique muscle, synapse in the "ciliary ganglion", and enter the eye as the "short posterior ciliary nerves" (Fig. 1.3B). Both divisions of

CN III pass through the annulus of Zinn into the muscle cone and innervate extraocular muscles from inside the muscle cone.

The sixth cranial nerve (CN VI), or "abducens nerve", innervates only the ipsilateral lateral rectus muscle. The fourth cranial nerve (CN IV), or "trochlear nerve", inner-vates only the superior oblique muscle. This nerve differs

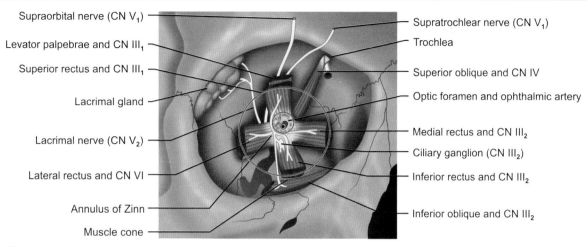

Fig. 1.2: Orbital nerves.
Source: Figure modified from Warwick R. Eugene Wolff's Anatomy of the Eye and Orbit. Philadelphia: WB Saunders Co;1977.

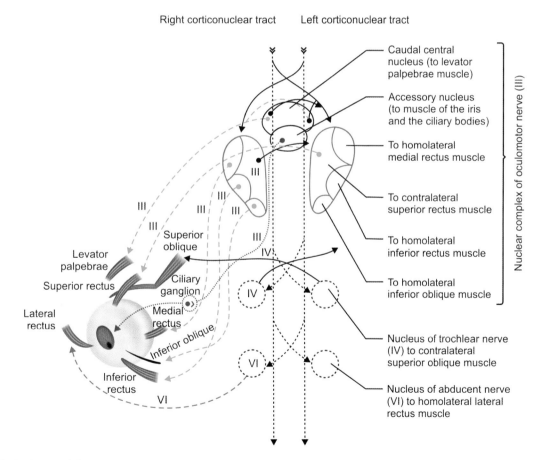

Fig. 1.3A: Brainstem nuclei.
Source: Figure modified from Grant JC: An Atlas of Anatomy. Baltimore: The Williams and Wilkins Co;1951.

from CN III and CN VI in not passing through the annulus of Zinn but rather innervating the superior oblique muscle from the orbital side. The fourth cranial nerve also differs by decussating and existing on the dorsal surface of the brainstem.

The "medial longitudinal fasciculus" (not shown) is a collection of fibers that interconnects these brainstem nuclei. The fasciculus passes medial to the abducens and lateral to the trochlear and oculomotor nuclei. The medial longitudinal fasciculus also connects these nuclei with the vestibular nuclei and is responsible for integrating conjugate movements of the eyes. A disruption of the fibers in this tract between CN VI and CN III results in a disconjugate movement of the eyes termed an "internuclear ophthalmoplegia" (see Chapter 13). In this disorder, there is a decreased ability of the ipsilateral eye to turn in on an attempted contralateral gaze.

The fifth cranial nerve (CN V) , or "trigeminal nerve", has only sensory branches in the orbit. The major branches from the first, or "ophthalmic, division" (CN V_1) are the "frontal" and "nasociliary nerves". The frontal nerve continues as the "supraorbital" and "supratrochlear nerves" to innervate the conjunctival and skin surfaces of the upper eyelid and forehead. The nasociliary nerve gives off two "long posterior ciliary nerves" subserving sensation to the eyeball and continues anteriorly to innervate the ethmoidal air cells and the anterolateral wall of the nose. From the second, or "maxillary, division" (CN V_2) the "infraorbital nerve" subserves sensation to both surfaces of the lower eyelid and the skin overlaying the maxilla, the side of the nose, and the lips. It also supplies sensory fibers to the lacrimal gland via the "lacrimal nerve". Parasympathetic lacrimal secretory fibers from the seventh cranial nerve (CN VII), or "facial nerve", travel with the lacrimal nerve after synapsing in the pterygopalatine ganglion, to innervate the lacrimal gland.

The "ophthalmic artery" is the first major branch of the internal carotid artery (Fig. 1.3B). Within the optic canal, it lies inferolateral to the optic nerve, but on entering the orbit it crosses over or under the nerve and runs medially. The first important intraorbital branch is the "central retinal artery", which enters the optic nerve about 12 mm behind the globe. As many as twenty "short posterior ciliary arteries" supplying the choroid and two "long posterior ciliary arteries" are also branches of the ophthalmic artery, as is the "lacrimal artery". Terminal branches of the

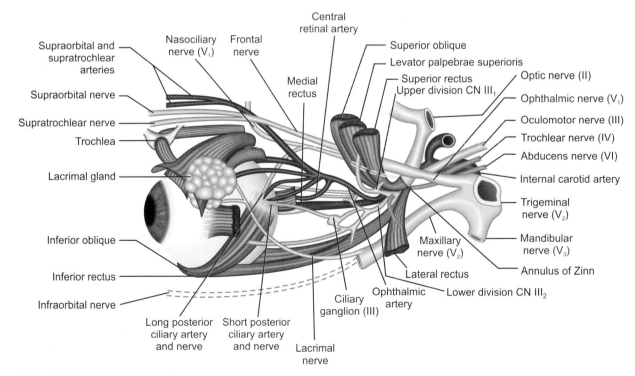

Fig. 1.3B: Orbital nerves and vessels.
Sources: Figure modified from Gray H, Lewis WH: Anatomy of the Human Body. Philadelphia: Lea & Febiger, 1918, and Grant JC: An Atlas of Anatomy. Baltimore: The Williams and Wilkins Co; 1951 and Bossy J. Atlas of Neuroanatomy and special sense organs. Philadelphia: WB Saunders Co; 1970.

ophthalmic artery include the "supraorbital", "supratrochlear" and "ethmoidal arteries". All the extraocular muscles are supplied by either the "lateral" or the "medial muscular branches" of the ophthalmic artery. From the branches supplying the rectus muscles arise the "anterior ciliary arteries". The latter anastomose with the long posterior ciliary arteries to supply the anterior globe. Venous drainage mirrors arterial supply except the major veins are located superiorly and inferiorly.

■ ORBITAL AND FASCIAL RELATIONSHIPS

The "periosteum" of the orbit unites posteriorly with the dura mater and the sheath of the optic nerve and is loosely adherent to the bones except at the bony sutures and apertures of the orbit. At the margin of the orbit, it fuses with the "orbital septum". The orbital septum attaches along the circumference of the orbit and covers the orbital surface of the base of the eyelids, separating the eyelids from the contents of the orbital cavity. In the upper eyelid, it fuses with the aponeurosis of the levator palpebrae superioris. At the medial and lateral corners of the eye, it attaches to the medial and lateral palpebral ligaments, respectively. Inferiorly, there is a similar relationship between the septum and the suspensory ligament of Lockwood (Figs 1.4 A and B).

"Tenon's capsule" is a smooth-surfaced elastic and fibrous tissue that envelops the globe and separates it from the orbital fat. It remains uncertain whether this capsule should be considered principally a socket, in which the eye rotates, or simply a fat barrier that moves with the globe. Tenon's capsule is perforated by the ciliary vessels and nerves, and fuses posteriorly with the optic nerve sheath. Anteriorly, it fuses with the bulbar conjunctiva to attach to the globe at the corneoscleral junction. The tendons of the extraocular muscles all must perforate Tenon's capsule to insert on the globe. At the site of penetration, the capsule fuses with the "muscle sheath". Prior to and after penetrating Tenon's capsule, the sheaths of the four rectus muscles spread out to form an "intermuscular membrane". Posterior to the globe the intermuscular membrane encases the muscle cone only for a short distance.

Additional fusions of the muscle sheaths are noteworthy. In the superior orbit, fusion of the sheaths of the superior rectus and levator muscles enhances their synergistic action. In the inferior orbit, the sheaths of the inferior rectus and inferior oblique fuse with each other and Tenon's capsule, forming a substantial band of fibrous tissue beneath the globe, which tapers upwardly to the medial and lateral rectus muscles. Because the latter have attachments to the orbital wall, it is thought that this suspension of fascia supports the globe like a hammock. This hammock-like band of tissue is called "Lockwood's ligament", although precisely which tissues constitute Lockwood's ligament are difficult to define. Typically included in the definition are extensions anterior to the fused inferior rectus and oblique

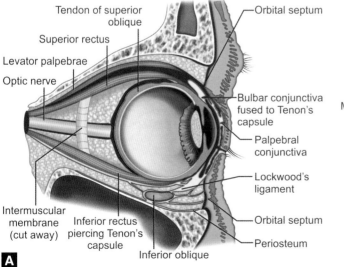

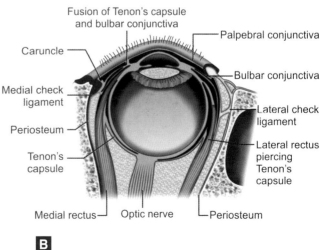

Figs 1.4A and B: Fascia of the eye. (A) Lateral view; (B) Superior view.
Source: (A) Figure modified from Gray H, Lewis WH: Anatomy of the Human Body. Philadelphia: Lea & Febiger, 1918. (B) Figure modified from Deaver JB: Surgical Anatomy of the Head and Neck. Philadelphia: P. Blakiston's son & Co;1904.

sheaths to the tarsal plate of the lower lid and the inferior orbital septum. Failure to separate these attachments during surgery of the inferior rectus can result in a change in the resting position of the lower lid.

Triangular extensions from the sheaths of the medial and lateral rectus muscles attach to the lacrimal and zygomatic bones, respectively. These expansions are strong and have been called "check ligaments", although it remains uncertain whether they actually limit eye movements.

The function of the fascial system is to support the globe and to allow smooth excursions of the eye. Essential to the integrity of the system is the elastic tissue septum attached to Tenon's capsule and the immovable periorbita. Inflammation that can result from laceration of the periorbita or Tenon's capsule converts elastic tissue to inelastic, resulting in restriction of ocular movement. Laceration of Tenon's capsule, with prolapse of extraconal fat into the sub-Tenon's capsule space, and the attendant inflammatory response are serious complications of strabismus surgery. These complications can result from blunt or careless sharp dissection of the muscle capsule or from searching for a rectus muscle beyond 10 mm from the limbus.

■ TOPOGRAPHIC ANATOMY OF THE GLOBE

Anterior to the equator of the globe, the four rectus muscles gently curve toward the eye to insert on the sclera at varying distances from the limbus (Fig. 1.5). Because the nasal aspect of the globe is closest to the orbital apex, the medial rectus muscle does not wrap around the globe as much as the other rectus muscles. Furthermore, the insertions of the "rectus muscles" are not equidistant from the limbus. The medial rectus inserts closest to the limbus followed sequentially by the inferior, lateral and superior rectus muscles. If one were to draw a line connecting the insertions of the rectus muscles, starting from the medial rectus, a spiral, termed the "spiral of Tillaux", would be formed. The insertions of the superior and inferior rectus muscles are curved slightly forward and obliquely. The nasal ends of their insertions are closer to the cornea than their temporal ends. The medial and lateral rectus muscles are more concentrically inserted.

Anterior to the rectus muscles, the "anterior ciliary arteries" emerge from the muscular branches of the ophthalmic artery. Two such arteries arise from each rectus muscle except for the lateral rectus muscle, from which there is only one.

The oblique muscles insert temporal to the vertical meridian of the eye, principally posterior to the equator (Figs 1.6 and 1.7). The obliquity of the insertion of the "superior oblique" causes the anterior edge to be closer to the limbus than the posterior edge. The anterior edge lies close to the temporal edge of the superior rectus. The "inferior oblique" muscle has either no tendon or a very

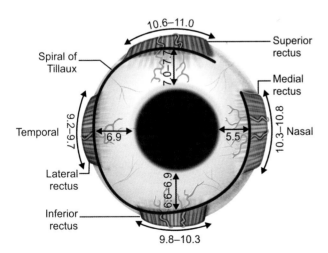

Fig. 1.5: Anterior view of the eye.
Source: Figure modified from Hogan MJ, Alvarado JA, Weddell JE. Histology of the Human Eye. Philadelphia: WB Saunders Co;1965.

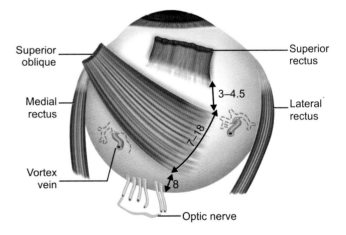

Fig. 1.6: Superior view of the eye.
Source: Figure modified from Hogan MJ, Alvarado JA, Weddell JE. Histology of the Human Eye. Philadelphia: WB Saunders Co;1965.

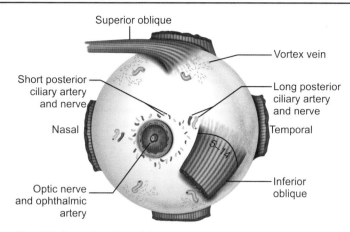

Fig. 1.7: Posterior view of the eye.
Source: Figure modified from Hogan MJ, Alvarado JA, Weddell JE. Histology of the Human Eye. Philadelphia: WB Saunders Co;1965.

short tendon. The medial border of its insertion lies close to the optic nerve and is about 2 mm below and temporal to the macula.

Posteriorly, about twenty "short posterior ciliary arteries" and eight "short posterior ciliary nerves" pierce the sclera around the optic nerve. Two "long posterior ciliary arteries" and "nerves" enter more distally along the horizontal meridian. Seven to eight "vortex veins" in each eye drain the venous system of the uveal tract. Their most common location is 3.0 mm posterior to the equator. Vortex veins exit on the temporal and medial aspects of the superior and inferior rectus muscles; these veins can be injured during surgery on the vertical recti or the oblique muscles.

■ BIBLIOGRAPHY

1. Bossy J. Atlas of Neuroanatomy and special sense organs. Philadelphia: WB Saunders Co;1970.
2. Hogan MJ, Alvarado JA, weddell JE. Histology of the Human Eye. Philadelphia: WB Saunders Co;1971.
3. Warwick R. Eugene Wolff's Anatomy of the Eye and orbit. Philadelphia: WB Saunders Co;1977.

2

Actions of the Extraocular Muscles

■ INTRODUCTION

The six extraocular muscles function to move the eye in the horizontal and vertical directions and to rotate the eye. Starting from a position with the eye and the head being directed straight ahead, termed the "primary position", the globe can be moved about 50° in each direction. Under normal conditions, however, such movement is not necessary, as the head will turn when the eyes are directed beyond 15–20° from the primary position.

The direction that a muscle turns an eye depends on the position of the eye in the orbit prior to the muscle's contraction. "Primary", "secondary" and "tertiary actions" of a muscle refer to the directions the eye is pulled, starting from the primary position. If the eye is placed in an eccentric position by the action of one muscle, contraction of a second muscle may result in a very different rotation of the eye than if the second muscle alone pulled the eye from the primary position.

A muscle will show its greatest effect when the axis of the muscle is in line with the optical axis of the eye. In testing the strength of muscles other than the horizontal recti, other muscles are always called on to rotate the eye away from the primary position so that the axis of the muscle in question is aligned with the optical axis. In testing the oblique muscles, the medial rectus is called on to turn the eye in so that the direction of pull of the oblique muscles is aligned with the optical axis. A similar relationship exists between the vertical recti and the lateral rectus muscle. Because the starting position of the eye is usually not the primary position when the strength of an individual muscle is tested, the primary, secondary and tertiary actions of a muscle do not necessarily correspond with the position of gaze used to test the strength of that muscle.

To describe the direction in which the eye is rotated on contracture of a specific extraocular muscle, it is convenient to discuss separately the horizontal rectus muscles, the vertical rectus muscles and the oblique muscles.

■ THE HORIZONTAL RECTUS MUSCLES

The medial and lateral rectus muscles (Fig. 2.1) are the only two extraocular muscles in which the muscle axis is aligned with the optical axis of the eye in the primary position. Because of this, the action of these muscles corresponds with the cardinal position of gaze used to test the strength of these muscles.

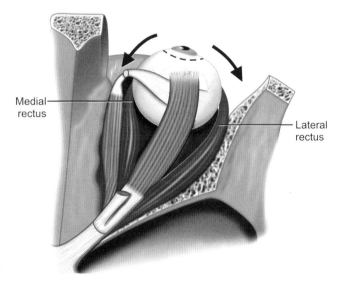

Fig. 2.1: The horizontal rectus muscles.

From the primary position, the action of the medial rectus muscle is solely to turn the eye in ("adduction"), and the action of the lateral rectus is to turn the eye out ("abduction").

■ THE VERTICAL RECTUS MUSCLES

When the eye is in the primary position, the vertical rectus muscles (Figs 2.2 to 2.4) form an angle of 23° with the optical axis. Because of this, the superior and inferior rectus muscles do not act solely to elevate or depress the eye when starting from the primary position. Contraction of a vertical rectus muscle from the primary position

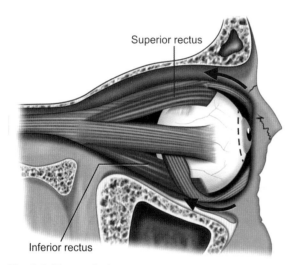

Fig. 2.2: The vertical rectus muscles.

adducts and cycloducts the eye. When the eye is turned out 23°, the optical axis of the eye is aligned with these muscle axes, and from this position principally vertical movement results from their contraction. As the eye turns in from this position, however, contraction of the vertical recti begins to cause adduction as well as cyclotorsion of the eye. The superior rectus causes incycloduction, and the inferior rectus brings about excycloduction. Theoretically, at 67° adduction the superior rectus would cause only incycloduction and adduction, and the inferior rectus excycloduction and adduction.

It is important to realize that from the primary position the superior rectus muscle elevates, adducts and incycloducts the eye (Fig. 2.5). To test the strength of this muscle, however, one would abduct the eye 23° to align the muscle axis with the optical axis to obtain the maximal vertical effect of superior rectus contraction (Fig. 2.6). From the primary position, the superior rectus adducts the eye, but the position of gaze necessary for testing its strength is the abducted position. The inferior rectus muscle is analogous except that the inferior rectus muscle depresses and excycloducts the eye from the primary position.

■ THE OBLIQUE MUSCLES

With the eye in the primary position, the superior oblique muscle forms an angle of 54° with the optical axis. From this position its primary action is to incycloduct the eye, but it also causes a small amount of abduction and depression. With the eye turned in 54° so that the axis of the tendon is aligned with the optical axis its vertical action becomes

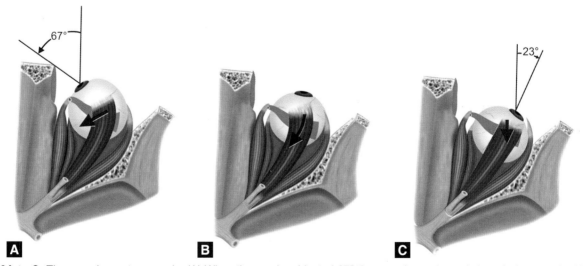

Figs 2.3A to C: The superior rectus muscle. (A) When the eye is adducted 67° the superior rectus only incycloducts and adducts the eye; (B) In primary position the superior rectus, elevates, adducts and incycloducts the eye; (C) When the eye is turned out 23°, the optical axis of the eye is aligned with the muscle axis. From this position the muscle primarily elevates the eye.

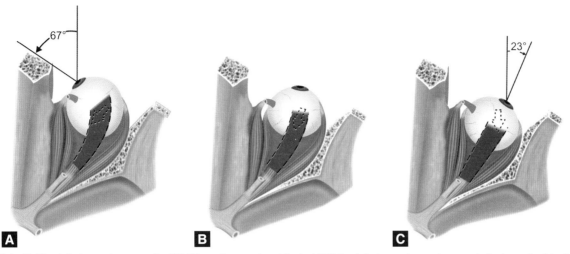

Figs 2.4A to C: The inferior rectus muscle. (A) When the eye is adducted 67° the inferior rectus only excycloducts and adducts the eye; (B) In primary position the inferior rectus, depresses, adducts and excycloducts the eye; (C) When the eye is turned out 23°, the optical axis of the eye is aligned with the muscle axis. From this position the muscle primarily depresses the eye.

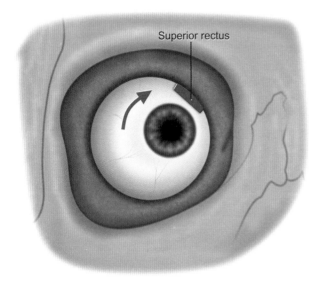

Fig. 2.5: Direction of rotation of eye from the primary position by the superior rectus muscle.

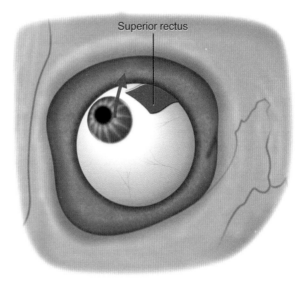

Fig. 2.6: Gaze position to test strength of superior rectus muscle.

pronounced. With the eye abducted, the superior oblique acts primarily to incycloduct and secondarily to abduct the eye (Figs 2.7A to C).

The inferior oblique muscle is similar to the superior oblique. With the eye in the primary position, the axis of this muscle forms an angle of 51° with the optical axis. From this position, its primary action is to excycloduct the eye, with secondary actions of abduction and elevation. With the eye adducted, the vertical action of the inferior oblique becomes pronounced. With the eye abducted, the inferior oblique acts primarily to excycloduct and secondarily to abduct the eye (Figs 2.8A to C).

In precise contrast to the vertical rectus muscles, the oblique muscles act to abduct the eye but strength of the oblique muscles is tested with the eye adducted. As shown for the superior oblique muscle (Fig. 2.9), from the primary position the superior oblique incycloducts, abducts and depresses the eye. With the eye starting in the adducted position, however, the tendon axis is aligned with the optical axis, and the maximal vertical action of the superior oblique can be brought out (Fig. 2.10).

Table 2.1 summarizes the primary, secondary and tertiary actions of the muscles when they are contracting with the eye in the primary position.

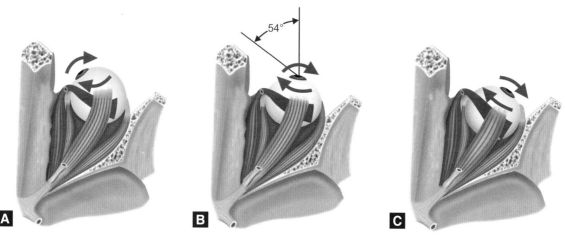

Figs 2.7A to C: The superior oblique muscle. (A) The vertical action of the muscle (depression of the eye) is pronounced when the eye is adducted; (B) With the eye in the primary position, the superior oblique muscle forms an angle of 54° with the optical axis. From this position its primary action is to incycloduct the eye, but it also causes a small amount of abduction and depression; (C) With the eye abducted, the superior oblique acts primarily to incycloduct and secondarily to abduct the eye.

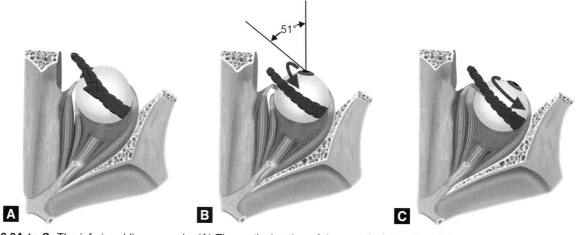

Figs 2.8A to C: The inferior oblique muscle. (A) The vertical action of the muscle (elevation of the eye) is pronounced when the eye is adducted; (B) With the eye in the primary position, the inferior oblique muscle forms an angle of 51° with the optical axis. From this position its primary action is to excycloduct the eye, but it also causes a small amount of abduction and elevation; (C) With the eye abducted, the inferior oblique acts primarily to excycloduct and secondarily to abduct the eye.

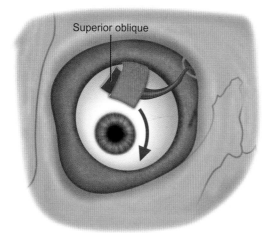

Fig. 2.9: Direction of rotation of eye from primary position by the superior oblique muscle.

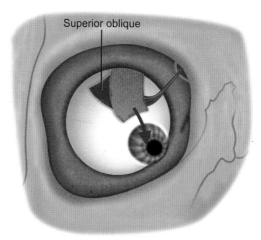

Fig. 2.10: Gaze position to test strength of the superior oblique muscle.

Table 2.1: Extraocular muscle actions with the eye in the primary position*

Muscle	Primary	Secondary	Tertiary
Medial rectus	Adduction	—	—
Lateral rectus	Abduction	—	—
Superior rectus	Elevation	Incycloduction	Adduction
Inferior rectus	Depression	Excycloduction	Adduction
Superior oblique	Incycloduction	Depression	Abduction
Inferior oblique	Excycloduction	Elevation	Abduction

*Vertical rectus muscles adduct the eye, but strength is tested with the eye abducted.
Oblique muscles abduct the eye, but strength is tested with the eye adducted.
Superior extraocular muscles incycloduct the eye.
Inferior extraocular muscles excycloduct the eye.

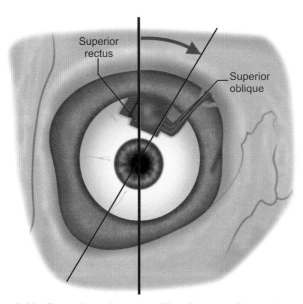

Fig. 2.11: From the primary position the superior rectus and superior oblique muscles incycloduct the eye.

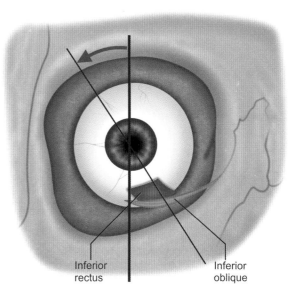

Fig. 2.12: From the primary position the inferior rectus and inferior oblique muscles excycloduct the eye.

■ INCYCLODUCTORS AND EXCYCLODUCTORS OF THE GLOBE

As a final note, it should be remembered that the superior muscles (superior rectus and superior oblique) incycloduct the eye (Fig. 2.11), whereas the inferior muscles (inferior rectus and inferior oblique) excycloduct the eye (Fig. 2.12). This is because the oblique muscles insert primarily posterior to the equator of the eye (see Figs 1.6 and 1.7).

■ BIBLIOGRAPHY

1. Demer JL. Current concepts of mechanical and neural factors in ocular motility. Curr Opin Neurol. 2006;19:4.
2. Jampel RS. The fundamental principle of the action of the oblique muscles. Am J Ophthalmol. 1970;69:623.
3. Mitchell PR, Parks MM. Eye movements and position. In: Tasman W, Jaeger EA (Eds). Clinical ophthalmology. Philadelphia: JB Lippincott Co;2013.
4. Warwick R, Williams PL. Gray's Anatomy. Philadelphia: WB Saunders Co;1973.

3

Physiology of Ocular Motility

■ THE CARDINAL POSITIONS OF GAZE

The insertion of each extraocular muscle is unique in both its location and the angle it subtends with the globe. For each muscle there is a singular position of the eye in which that muscle alone has a mechanical advantage and will act as the primary mover of the eye. There are six extraocular muscles; therefore, six such positions called the "cardinal positions of gaze" exist (Fig. 3.1). Because each position is unique for a given muscle, the strength of a muscle can be tested by asking the patient to look in

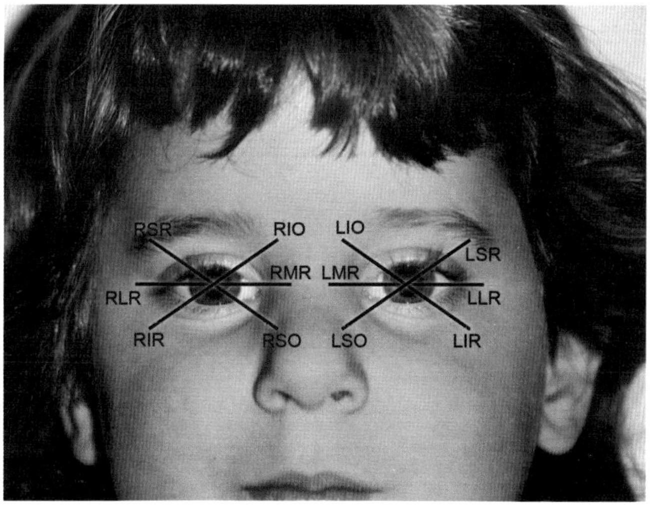

Fig. 3.1: Primary muscles that act in the six cardinal positions of gaze for each eye. *RSR: Right superior rectus; RLR: Right lateral rectus; RIR: Right inferior rectus; RSO: Right superior oblique; RMR: Right medial rectus: RIO: Right inferior oblique; LIO: Left inferior oblique; LMR: Left medial rectus; LSO: Left superior oblique; LIR: Left inferior rectus; LLR: Left lateral rectus; LSR: Left superior rectus.

the direction of the muscle's individual cardinal position. The cardinal positions of gaze are determined by having the muscles contract for maximal vertical or horizontal effect by aligning the muscle and the optical axes. Table 3.1 summarizes the muscles that act in the six cardinal positions of gaze for each eye.

It is important to know the distinction between the actions of a muscle and the cardinal positions of gaze. The primary, secondary and tertiary actions of a muscle describe the movement of the eye when the muscle contracts with the eye in the primary position (see Chapter 2). With the exception of the horizontal rectus muscles, the directions the eye is pulled by the actions of a muscle (from the primary position) do not correspond to the cardinal position in which the eye is placed to test the strength of that muscle.

Table 3.1: Conjugate movements of the eyes into the cardinal positions of gaze	
Movement	*Responsible Muscles**
Up and right	RSR and LIO
Straight right	RLR and LMR
Down and right	RIR and LSO
Down and left	RSO and LIR
Straight left	RMR and LLR
Up and left	RIO and LSR

*RSR: Right superior rectus; RLR: Right lateral rectus; RIR: Right inferior rectus; RSO: Right superior oblique; RMR: Right medial rectus: RIO: Right inferior oblique; LIO: Left inferior oblique; LMR: Left medial rectus; LSO: Left superior oblique; LIR: Left inferior rectus; LLR: Left lateral rectus; LSR: Left superior rectus

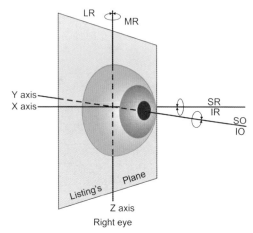

Fig. 3.2: The three primary axes of Fick [vertical (Z), horizontal (X), and anteroposterior (Y)] and the muscles that control movement about each of these axes for the right eye. *LR: Lateral rectus; MR: Medial rectus; SR: Superior rectus; IR: Inferior rectus; SO: Superior oblique; IO: Inferior oblique.

Table 3.2: Agonist synergist and antagonist relationships			
Position	*Agonist*	*Synergists*	*Antagonists*
Adduction	Medial rectus	Superior rectus Inferior rectus	Lateral rectus Superior oblique Inferior oblique
Abduction	Lateral rectus	Superior oblique Inferior oblique	Medial rectus Superior rectus Inferior rectus
Elevation	Superior rectus	Inferior oblique	Inferior rectus Superior oblique
Depression	Inferior rectus	Superior oblique	Superior rectus Inferior oblique
Incycloduction	Superior oblique	Superior rectus	Inferior oblique Inferior rectus
Excycloduction	Inferior oblique	Inferior rectus	Superior oblique Superior rectus

■ MONOCULAR EYE MOVEMENTS

Agonist and Antagonist Relationships

The actions of the extraocular muscles are exquisitely balanced. Fick[1] first noted that any movement of the eye can be described as a rotation about a vertical (Z), a horizontal (X), or an anteroposterior (Y) axis; these axes have come to be known as the three "primary axes of Fick" (Fig. 3.2). Horizontal movements occur about the Z axis, vertical about the X axis, and torsional about the Y axis. The X and Z axes constitute the two-dimensional "Listing's plane", the center of which is the center of ocular rotation.

Ocular motility is so finely balanced that the six muscles of the eye can be divided into three pairs; each pair controls movement about one of the axes of Fick. As shown in Figure 3.2, the two muscles in each pair oppose each other. The primary muscle that moves an eye in a given direction (e.g. rotation upward about the X axis performed by the superior rectus) is called the "agonist". The muscle that opposes the action of the agonist (in this instance the inferior rectus) is called an "antagonist". The "synergist" is the muscle that acts in concert with the agonist to produce a given movement. Table 3.2 summarizes agonist, antagonist and synergist relationships.

Sherrington's Law

"Sherrington's law of reciprocal innervation" describes the relationship between an agonist and an antagonist during normal movement of the eye. It states that stimulation of a muscle to contract is accompanied by inhibition of contraction of its antagonists.[2] On abduction of the right eye (Fig. 3.3) the right lateral rectus muscle is stimulated while the right medial rectus muscle is inhibited. Sherrington's law, applying as it does to agonist and antagonist muscles, describes a **monocular** phenomenon concerning the actions of muscles in an **individual** eye. Exceptions to this law are responsible for the aberrant ocular movements seen in some pathologic conditions. Two important examples are "Duane's retraction syndrome", in which co-contraction of the medial and lateral rectus muscles of the same eye occurs, and "Parinaud's syndrome", in which rhythmic contractions of the medial and lateral rectus muscles (retraction nystagmus) occurs on attempted upward gaze (see Chapter 13).

Ductions

"Ductions" are monocular eye movements about one of the axes of Fick. Appropriate prefixes define the direction in which the eye is rotating. "Abduction" is movement of the eye temporally (Fig. 3.3) and "adduction" is movement nasally (Fig. 3.4), both of which occur about the Z axis. "Supraduction" is upward rotation (Fig. 3.5), "infraduction" is downward rotation (Fig. 3.6), and both occur about the X axis. "Excycloduction" (extorsion) is defined as temporal rotation of the 12:00 meridian of the cornea (Fig. 3.7; also see Fig. 2.12), and "incycloduction" (intorsion) is a nasal rotation of the 12:00 meridian of the cornea (Fig. 3.8; also see Fig. 2.11), both of which occur about the Y axis.

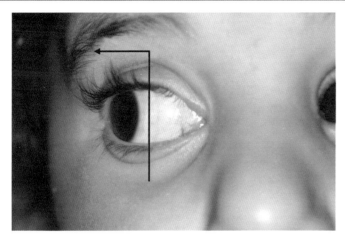

Fig. 3.3: Abduction of the right eye.

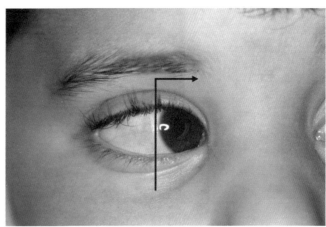

Fig. 3.4: Adduction of the right eye.

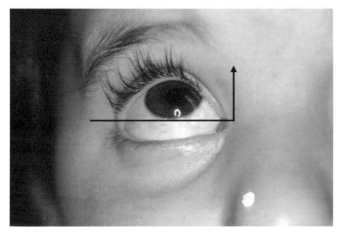

Fig. 3.5: Supraduction of the right eye.

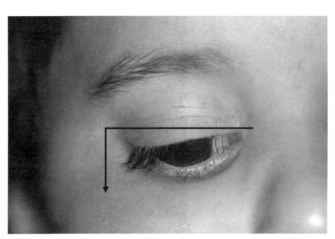

Fig. 3.6: Infraduction of the right eye.

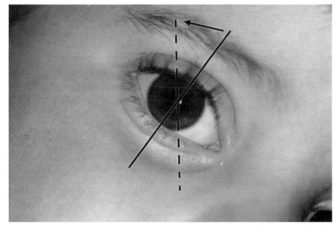

Fig. 3.7: Excycloduction of the right eye.

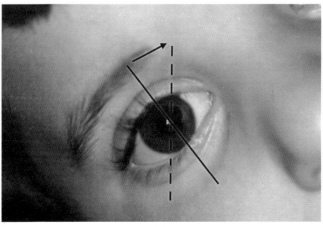

Fig. 3.8: Incycloduction of the right eye.

■ BINOCULAR EYE MOVEMENTS

Ductions describe monocular movements, and agonists and antagonists refer to different muscles in the same eye that act in concert or against each other. Different terms are used to describe movements of the two eyes together, and a special term, "yoke muscles", is given to the corresponding muscles of the two eyes that affect movement of both eyes into a specific gaze position. The muscle pairs listed in Table 3.1 that turn the eyes into the six cardinal positions of gaze are yoke muscles.

Versions

Any movements of the two eyes in the same direction at the same time and of approximately the same magnitude are called "conjugate movements". "Versions" are conjugate binocular eye movements brought about by contraction of yoke muscles. "Dextroversion" is movement of both eyes to the right (Fig. 3.9), and "levoversion" is movement to the left (Fig. 3.10). Elevation of both eyes is called "supraversion" (Fig. 3.11), and depression is called "infraversion" (Fig. 3.12). "Levocycloversion" is rotation of both eyes so that the 12:00 meridian of each cornea is rotated to the left (Fig. 3.13), and "dextrocycloversion" is a rotation to the right of the 12:00 meridian of each cornea (Fig. 3.14).

Vergences

"Vergences" are binocular movements in which the eyes move in opposite directions, or "disjugately". "Convergence" is the nasal rotation of each eye (Fig. 3.15), and "divergence" is temporal rotation (Fig. 3.16). "Positive vertical divergence" (right sursumvergence) occurs when the right eye moves up while the left eye moves down (Fig. 3.17). "Negative vertical divergence" (right deorsumvergence) is the opposite movement (Fig. 3.18). "Incyclovergence" (conclination) occurs when the 12:00 meridian of both eyes rotates nasally (Fig. 3.19). "Excyclovergence" (disclination) is temporal rotation of both eyes (Fig. 3.20).

Hering's Law

"Hering's law" is the law of yoke muscles, pertaining to binocular eye movements. When one muscle in a pair of yoke muscles is stimulated the other is simultaneously and equally stimulated.[3] Similarly, inhibition of a muscle is associated with inhibition of its yoke. This law applies to all voluntary and some involuntary eye movements. On dextroversion (Fig. 3.21), the right lateral rectus and its yoke, the left medial rectus, are stimulated while the yoked right medial and left lateral rectus muscles are inhibited, as confirmed electromyographically (Fig. 3.22). Yoke pairs change for disjugate or vergence movements, and with convergence both medial rectus muscles contract while the lateral rectus muscles relax (Figs 3.23 and 3.24). On head tilt, the vestibular ocular reflex causes rotation of the eyes in a direction opposite the head tilt to keep the eyes aligned vertically. Sherrington's law describes the antagonist relationship between the incycloductors and excycloductors of a given eye, whereas Hering's law describes the relationship between the two eyes that allows both eyes to move conjugately and rotate together opposite the head tilt (Figs 3.25 and 3.26). An exception to Hering's law is "dissociated vertical deviation" (DVD) which can occur in congenital esotropia (see Chapter 8).

Clinical Applications of Hering's Law

According to Hering's law, the amount of innervation going to corresponding yoke muscles to achieve a desired position of gaze is the same. In paralytic strabismus, a paretic muscle will not contract as well as its yoke, which receives the same innervation, causing a misalignment of the eyes. Excessive stimulation is needed for fixation with a paretic muscle in its field of action. The excessive innervation causes the ocular misalignment to be greater when the paretic muscle fixates. The "primary deviation" is the deviation of the paretic eye with the sound eye fixating. The "secondary deviation" is the deviation of the sound eye when the eye with the paretic muscle is fixating. As noted, the secondary deviation is always greater than the primary deviation.

The patient that is the subject of Figures 3.27 to 3.29 has a paretic right superior rectus muscle and demonstrates the distinction between primary and secondary deviations. When she fixates a fixed object above her, equal innervation goes to both superior recti, according to Hering's law. When she fixates with her sound left superior rectus muscle (Fig. 3.27) a small right hypotropia

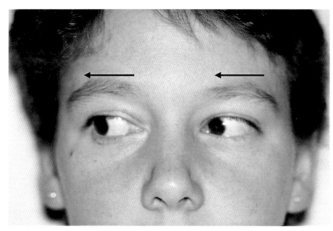

Fig. 3.9: Dextroversion.

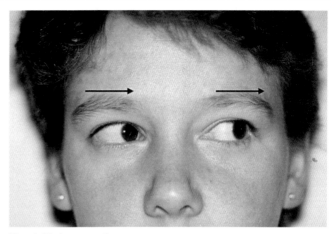

Fig. 3.10: Levoversion.

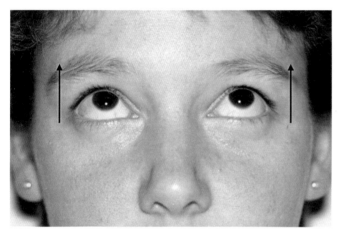

Fig. 3.11: Supraversion (elevation).

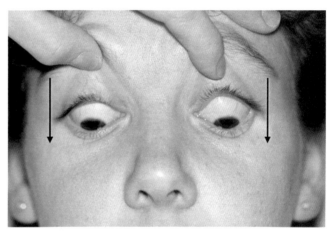

Fig. 3.12: Infraversion (depression).

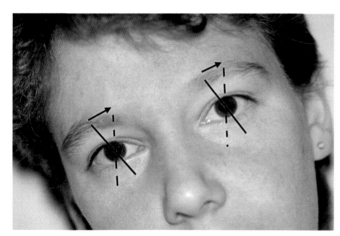

Fig. 3.13: Levocylcoversion.

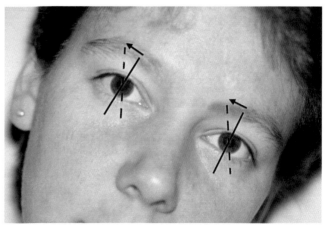

Fig. 3.14: Dextrocycloversion.

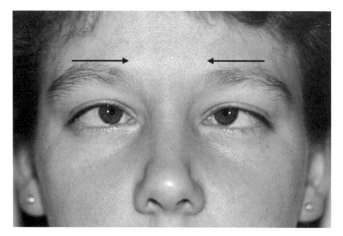

Fig. 3.15: Convergence.

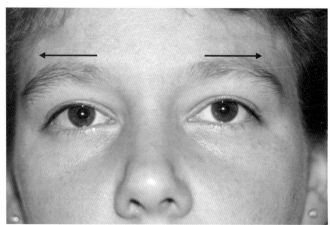

Fig. 3.16: Divergence.

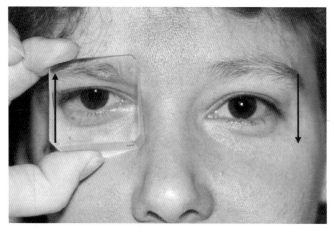

Fig. 3.17: Positive vertical divergence (right sursumvergence).

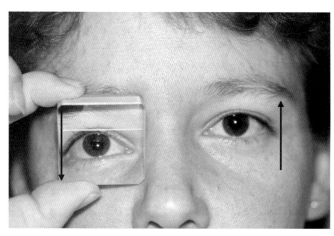

Fig. 3.18: Negative vertical divergence (right deorsumvergence).

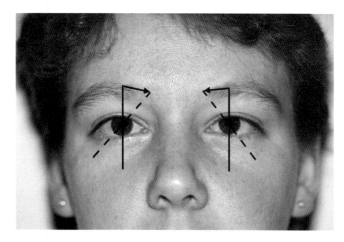

Fig. 3.19: Incyclovergence (conclination).

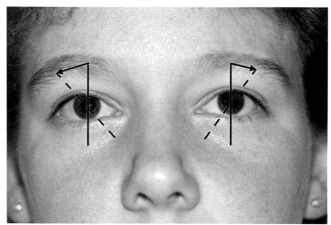

Fig. 3.20: Excyclovergence (disclination).

(the primary deviation) is evident (Fig 3.28). In order to fixate with the right eye, excessive stimulation of the right superior rectus is needed, which in turn leads to excessive stimulation of the left superior rectus (Fig. 3.29). The hypotropia of the right eye with the paretic right eye fixating (the secondary deviation) is larger (Fig. 3.30). In paralytic strabismus, the greater the stimulation is, the greater the misalignment becomes.

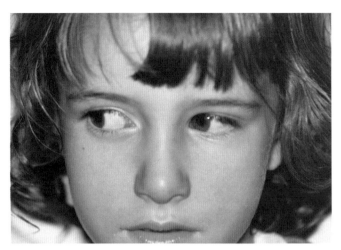

Fig. 3.21: Dextroversion.

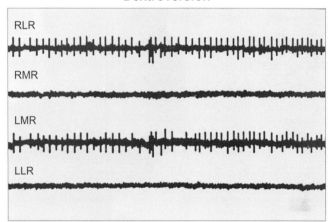

Fig. 3.22: Electromyograph of individual in Figure 3.21. On dextroversion the right lateral rectus (RLR) and its yoke the left medial rectus (LMR) are stimulated, and the yoked right medial rectus (RMR) and left lateral rectus (LLR) muscles are inhibited.

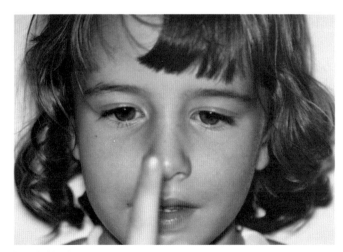

Fig. 3.23: Convergence.

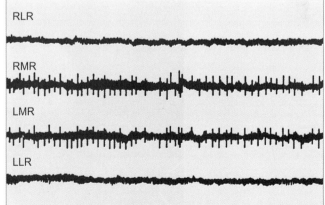

Fig. 3.24: Electromyograph of individual in Figure 3.23 demonstrating that yoke pairs change with disjugate movements. On convergence both medial rectus muscles contract while the lateral rectus muscles relax. (RLR: Right lateral rectus; RMR: Right medial rectus; LMR: Left medial rectus; LLR: Left lateral rectus).

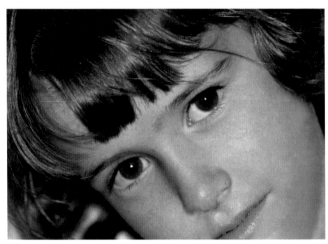

Fig. 3.25: Levocycloversion upon tilting the head to the right.

Levocycloversion

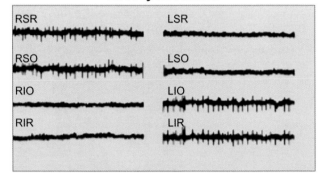

Fig. 3.26: Electromyograph of individual in Figure 3.25 demonstrating both Sherrington's and Herring's laws. According to Sherrington's law the incycloductors the right eye contract while the excycloductors of the same eye relax. According to Herring's law, simultaneous with the actions in the right eye, in the left eye the excycloductors contract and the incycloductors relax. (RSR: Right superior rectus; RSO: Right superior oblique; RIO: Right inferior oblique; RIR: Right inferior rectus; LSR: Left superior rectus; LSO: Left superior oblique; LIO: Left inferior oblique; LIR: Left inferior rectus)

Fixating with left eye

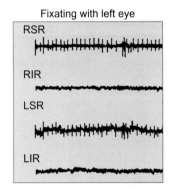

Fig. 3.27: Electromyograph of a patient with a right superior rectus muscle palsy fixating on an object above her with her sound left superior rectus muscle. (RSR: Right superior rectus; RIR: Right inferior rectus; LSR: Left superior rectus; LIR: Left inferior rectus).

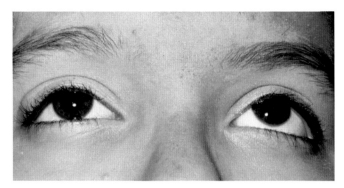

Fig. 3.28: A patient with a right superior rectus (RSR) muscle palsy fixating on an object above her with her sound left superior rectus muscle. The primary deviation is a small right hypotropia.

Fixating with right eye

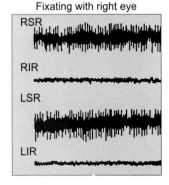

Fig. 3.29: Electromyograph of the patient with paretic right superior rectus muscle fixating on an object above her with her paretic right superior rectus muscle. Note the excessive stimulation of both the right and left superior rectus muscles. (RSR: Right superior rectus; RIR: Right inferior rectus; LSR: Left superior rectus; LIR: Left inferior rectus).

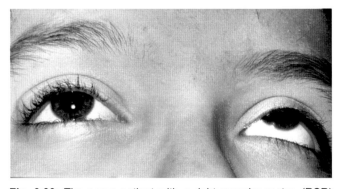

Fig. 3.30: The same patient with a right superior rectus (RSR) muscle palsy fixating on an object above her with her paretic right superior rectus muscle. The secondary deviation is a larger right hypotropia.

■ REFERENCES

1. Fick A. Neue Versuche über die Augenstellung. Moleschott's Unters. 1858;5:193.
2. Sherrington CS. Experimental note on two movements of the eyes. J Physiol (Lond). 1894;17:27.
3. Hering E. Die Lehre vom Binocularen Sehen. Leipzig: Wilhelm Engelmann;1868.

■ BIBLIOGRAPHY

1. Alpern M. Movements of the eyes. In: Davson H (Ed). The Eye, volume 3. New York: Academic Press; 1962.
2. von Noorden GK, Campos EC. Binocular vision and ocular motility. 6th edition. St Louis, Mo: CV Mosby; 2002.

Sensory Physiology and Pathology

VISUAL ACUITY

Amblyopia

The assessment of visual acuity is essential to any ocular evaluation and is especially important in the strabismic child in order to detect amblyopia. "Amblyopia" (Greek, "dull vision") is a deficiency of corrected central visual acuity in the absence of a structural abnormality of the fovea. Characteristics and categories of this disorder are summarized in Table 4.1.

Amblyopia affects approximately 2.0–2.5% of the general population. It can result from any condition that prevents a clear image from being focused on the retina. Treatment of the inciting condition, such as removing a congenital cataract or straightening a misaligned eye, does not cure the amblyopia. In addition to optically correcting the affected eye, treatment involves stimulating the fovea of the eye by preventing visual input to the other eye. This is done through occluding the nonamblyopic eye with a patch (Fig. 4.1), an occluder behind glasses (Fig. 4.2), a neutral density filter behind glasses (Figs 4.3 and 4.4), or other optical means.

Measuring Visual Acuity in the Preverbal Child

The "fixation response" is a reliable and easily performed assessment of vision in the preverbal child. The ability of each eye to attain and maintain fixation on a movable small object is tested by simply occluding the other eye. The response can be graded as to whether fixation is central and steady and is maintained when the occluder is removed from the other eye (Figs 4.5A and B). The ability to generate "optokinetic nystagmus" (OKN) using an OKN

Table 4.1: Amblyopia
Characteristics
• May be unilateral or bilateral
• Visual acuity worse when reading a row as opposed to individual symbols (the crowding phenomenon)
• Less reduction of acuity when looking through a neutral density filter than in eyes with organic macular disease
• Relative afferent pupillary defect not usually seen unless amblyopia is very dense
• Fixation with amblyopic eye may be eccentric (nonfoveal)
Categories
• *Strabismic*: Usually unilateral; results from prolonged and continual fixation by one eye and suppression of images from the other
• *Refractive*: Associated with large hyperopic, myopic, or astigmatic errors
• *Anisometropic*: Subtype of above when amblyopia occurs only in the more ametropic eye
• *Deprivation (amblyopia ex-anopsia)*: Occurs when a focused image cannot be formed on the retina because of an obstruction in the visual axis

drum, as shown in Figure 4.6, is another easily performed test of visual function.

Several techniques have been refined in an attempt to objectively evaluate visual function in preverbal children. The two techniques of greatest interest are tests of preferential looking (PL) and visual evoked potentials (VEP). "Preferential looking" is based on the observation that infants prefer to fixate a patterned stimuli (usually a grating is used) rather than a homogeneous field. Various series of gratings are presented to the child, and acuity is estimated by determining the smallest grating that the

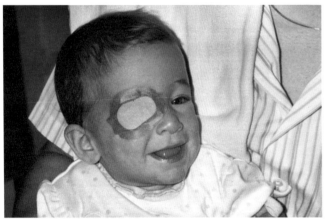

Fig. 4.1: Occlusion of a non-amblyopic eye with an eye-patch.

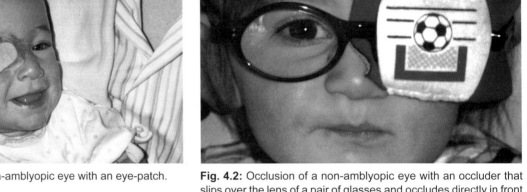

Fig. 4.2: Occlusion of a non-amblyopic eye with an occluder that slips over the lens of a pair of glasses and occludes directly in front as well as to the side of the glasses.

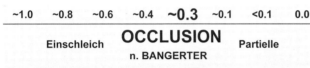

| ~1.0 | ~0.8 | ~0.6 | ~0.4 | ~0.3 | ~0.1 | <0.1 | 0.0 |

OCCLUSION

Einschleich   n. BANGERTER   Partielle

Montage:

1. Occlusive-Folien auf Glasform – 1 mm kleiner – zuschnel-den.
2. Glanzseite der Folie und Brillenglas reinigen, entfetten.
3. Folie auf ganz nasse Innenseite des Glases andrücken, trocknen bis keine Luftblase mehr sichtbar ist.

Montage:

1. Couper la feuille d' occlusion à la forme du verre de la lunette – moins un millimetre.
2. Nettoyer et dégraisser le verre et la feuille.
3. Appliquer la côté brillant de la feuille sur la face intérieure du verre bien trempé, sécher. – Aucune bulle d'air doît rester visible.

Application instructions:

1. Cut foil 1 mm smaller than spectacle glass.
2. Wash glass thoroughly. Wet glossy side of foil.
3. Apply glossy side of foil to the still wet inside of glass. Press with dry cloth. Rub to remove all bubbles.

Fig. 4.3: Instructions for applying a neutral density filter to the inside surface of the non-amblyopic eye's eyeglass lens.

infant will preferentially fixate. Older children can point to the side with the gratings (Fig. 4.7). "Visual evoked potentials" measure the electrophysiologic response of the visual cortex when the child is presented with either phase-alternated checkerboards or square-wave gratings (Fig. 4.8).

Measuring Visual Acuity in the Verbal Child and Adult

The measurement of visual acuity in the literate child or adult involves the use of standard letters originally designed by Snellen. An entire Snellen letter when viewed from 20 feet subtends an angle of 5 minutes of arc at the

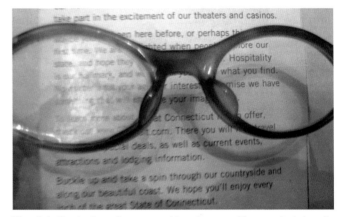

Fig. 4.4: Occlusion of a non-amblyopic eye with a neutral density filter applied to the inside of the right lens of a pair of glasses. Notice that the neutral density filter is barely visible.

nodal point of the eye. Each of the respective elements of the letter subtends an angle of 1 minute of arc (Fig. 4.9).

Typically, a "Snellen acuity chart" is made up of rows of letters of gradually decreasing size as one descends the chart (Fig. 4.10). Acuity is usually recorded as an unreduced fraction based on a normal viewing distance of 20 feet. The numerator of the fraction is the viewing distance, and the denominator represents the distance at which a normal emmetropic observer should be able to resolve the same size letter. Criticisms of the standard Snellen chart include the wide variation in difficulty of the letters used, the irregular progression of letter size, and the different number of letters and spacing of letters on each line. Charts have been developed using an equal number of Sloan letters of approximately equal difficulty on each line, with a geometric progression of letter height from line to line (Fig. 4.11). These charts are called "Log MAR charts" because they are based on a logarithmic scale of the minimal angle of resolution.

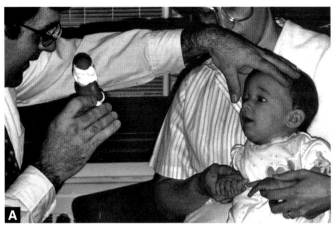

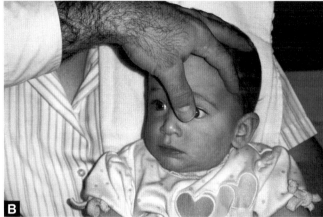

Figs 4.5A and B: (A) Testing fixation of left eye by occluding the right eye and (B) right eye by occluding the left eye.

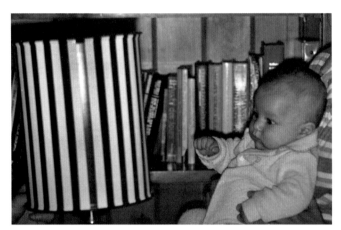

Fig. 4.6: Testing visual function with an optokinetic drum. Slow rotation of the drum in one direction will elicit optokinetic nystagmus with the fast movement of the eyes in the opposite direction.

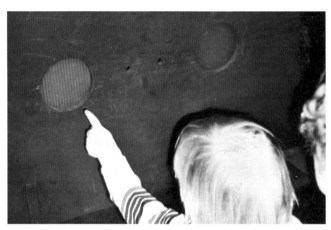

Fig. 4.7: Older preverbal child pointing to the side with the grating during preferential looking test.
Courtesy: John W Simon.

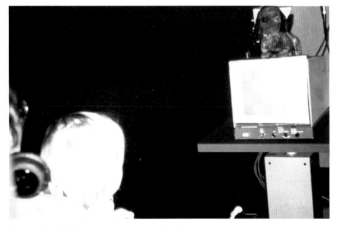

Fig. 4.8: Child being tested with for visual evoked potentials by being presented a phase-alternating checkerboard pattern on a monitor.
Courtesy: John W Simon.

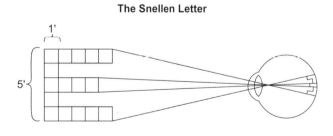

Fig. 4.9: The Snellen "E" letter. When viewed from 20 feet the entire letter subtends five minutes of arc at the nodal point of the eye and each of the elements of the letter subtend one minute of arc.

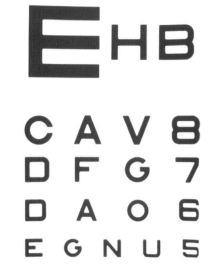

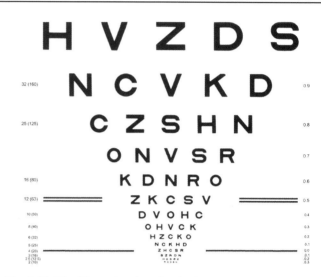

Fig. 4.10: The Snellen visual acuity chart.

Fig. 4.11: The Sloan visual acuity chart.

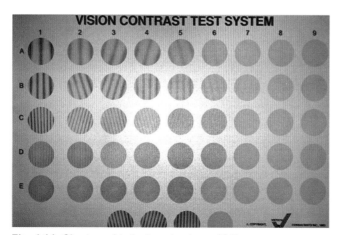

Fig. 4.12: "Picture" chart used to test the visual acuity of a child.

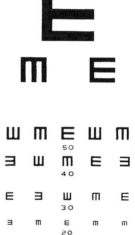

Fig. 4.13: "Illiterate E" chart used to test the visual acuity of a child.

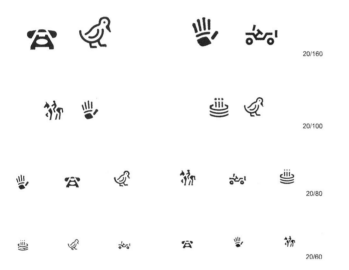

Fig. 4.14: Chart used to test contrast sensitivity.

For children various "picture charts" (Fig. 4.12), an "illiterate "E" chart" (Fig. 4.13), and a "Londholt broken ring" chart have been developed. Illiterate patients are asked to indicate the orientation of the "E" or the ring.

"Contrast sensitivity threshold tests" (Fig. 4.14) assess a parameter of the visual system not tested with the usual Snellen acuity tests. They may be helpful in patients with optic neuritis, glaucoma, diabetic retinopathy, and compressive lesions of the optic nerve and chiasm. Differences in contrast sensitivity in anisometropic and deprivation amblyopia have also been noted.

BINOCULAR VISION

The sensory physiology of the eye can most easily be understood by realizing that in a patient with two functioning eyes one of three physiologic sensory states must exist. The patient may have "no binocular vision", in which case only one or the other eye is used at any given time; completely "normal binocular vision" with a fine ability to appreciate depth; or some intermediate state. All the sensory adaptations to strabismus pertain to this intermediate state and occur in response to an acquired misalignment of the eyes in children who had previously developed normal binocular vision. The study of sensory adaptations to strabismus requires an understanding of what constitutes normal binocular vision and how the visual system adapts to retain some binocular vision when the eyes become misaligned. It does not deal with the uncorrected, congenitally esotropic patient who never developed binocular vision or with any patient with monocular vision.

Binocular vision begins to develop by 6 months of age in the infant with aligned eyes and focused retinal images and results in the blending or fusing of separate images from the two eyes into a single mental image. In its most developed form, this blending of images results in the ability to appreciate the third dimension of space, the perception of depth (stereopsis).

Parks divided binocular vision into two separate entities that he called "macular binocular vision" (MBV) and "extramacular binocular vision" (EBV).[1] Table 4.2 summarizes the characteristics of each. Macular binocular vision is necessary for what is generally known as "normal binocular vision" and excellent appreciation of depth. Whenever MBV is present EBV always coexists, but the reverse may not be true. Macular binocular vision is responsible for the fine perception of depth, but it is a tenuous, easily lost system that requires continual reinforcement. Adaptability in MBV does not exist. Extramacular binocular vision allows only gross depth perception because it is a function of peripheral retinal elements. The importance of EBV lies in its easy adaptability and tenacity in childhood to retain some binocularity and sensory fusion when the eyes become misaligned.

NORMAL BINOCULAR VISION (MACULAR BINOCULAR VISION)

Objective and Subjective Visual Directions

The act of seeing involves both objective and subjective aspects. "Objective visual direction" describes the path of reflected light from objects in the environment through the optics of the eye to the retina. "Subjective visual direction" describes the conscious awareness of where objects are localized in space. Normally, the two coincide.

A line drawn from an object in space through the nodal point of the eye to the retinal element it will stimulate represents the "line of direction" of the object. Each retinal element has a spatial value and will localize in space where an object must lie if it is stimulated.

The Object of Regard and Corresponding Retinal Points

Each retinal element has a visual direction slightly different from any other element of that retina. The coordinate use of the two eyes, however, requires that there be retinal elements in the two eyes that have the same visual direction.

Table 4.2 Binocular vision	
Macular Binocular Vision	*Extramacular Binocular Vision*
• No simultaneous perception of disparate images (physiologic suppression; retinal rivalry)	• Simultaneous perception of disparate images (confusion)
• Minimal fusional amplitudes to retinal image disparity	• Large fusional amplitudes to fuse disparate images
• Tolerant of deviation up to two thirds of a prism diopter	• Tolerant of deviation up to 8 prism diopters
• Excellent stereopsis possible (14–50 seconds of arc)	• Gross stereopsis only (60–3000 seconds of arc)
• Tenuous, easily lost system	• Fastidious system
• *Requires*: no strabismus; equal visual input; minimal anisometropia	• *Tolerates*: up to about 8 prism diopters of deviation; moderate anisometropia
• Adaptability does not exist or ceases to exist in absence of ideal situations; requires continual reinforcement	• Very adaptable in children (suppression and anomalous retinal correspondence develop)
• Always coexists with extramacular binocular vision	• May exist without macular binocular vision

These points are called "corresponding retinal points", and when stimulated give rise to the perception of the same visual direction. The foveas are the most important corresponding retinal points because they are the site of sharpest acuity. Furthermore, fixation of objects by the foveas provides the sensation of looking directly at an object; this object becomes the "object of regard" (Fig. 4.15), from which all other objects are referenced.

The Horopter

In the absence of misaligned eyes the fovea of one eye will always be the corresponding retinal point of the other eye, and both will be directed toward the object of regard. At any given distance, there will be points to either side of the object of regard whose images fall on corresponding retinal points and are perceived as a single image. If one connects these points in space, the two-dimensional structure that is constructed is called a "horopter" (Fig. 4.16). An infinite number of horopters can be constructed at an infinite number of fixation distances of the object of regard.

The foveas will always be corresponding retinal points, but other corresponding points change, depending on the distance of the object of regard. In Figure 4.17, two horopters are constructed for different distances of the object of regard. In both, the foveas are corresponding points. For the nearer horopter, *a* in the left eye corresponds with *a* in the right eye. For the more distant horopter, *a* in the left eye corresponds with *a¢* in the right eye.

The horopter has a curved surface, but each place on the horopter will be perceived as being exactly the same distance from the observer. Points nearer the end of the curve will actually lie closer to the observer, but as a consequence of corresponding retinal points, the two eyes function and reference objects as if the individual had only one eye located between the two. This concept has been termed the "cyclopean eye".

Panum's Fusional Space

When noncorresponding retinal points of the two eyes are stimulated by the same object, diplopia results. Panum discovered that there is a zone about the horopter where slightly disparate, noncorresponding retinal points stimulated by the same object can be fused and seen as single.[2] Near the fovea, only a slight degree of disparity is tolerated before diplopia results, but as one approaches peripheral retinal elements, ever increasing amounts of retinal disparity can be fused. It is common practice to mark a zone in front of or behind the horopter, in which an

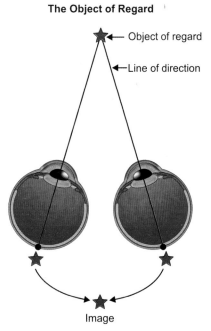

Fig. 4.15: Fixation of an object by an individual without strabismus or amblyopia. Because the image of the object strikes the fovea of each eye it produces the sensation of looking directly at the object. This object becomes the "Object of Regard".

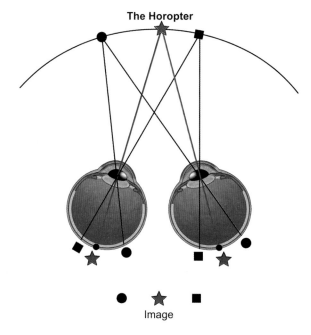

Fig. 4.16: The Horopter is a two-dimensional structure consisting of all of the points in space whose images fall on corresponding retinal points when the eyes are fixating on a specific object (the Object of Regard).

object may lie and still be seen as a single image despite stimulating noncorresponding retinal elements. This zone has been termed "Panum's fusional space". In reality, the physiologic basis to Panum's fusional space lies in the retina. As shown in Figure 4.18, retinal correspondence is not precisely point for point. Instead, a roughly circular zone of one retina corresponds to each retinal point of the opposite eye. These areas, in which fusion of disparate images of the same object occurs, are very small near the fovea but increase in size as one approaches the retinal periphery.

Physiologic Diplopia

Any object that lies outside of Panum's fusional space will form images on noncorresponding retinal points that are so disparate that they cannot be fused and are therefore seen as double. This is the basis of "physiologic diplopia" (Fig. 4.19). Objects located proximal to Panum's fusional space form images on temporal retina and are seen as closer as well as double. Objects located distal to Panum's space form images on nasal retina and are seen as further away as well as double. The distance between the double

images is a function of how far from Panum's space the object lies. The farther from Panum's space the object lies, the more widely separated the two images are. One is not generally aware of physiologic diplopia because the images strike nonfoveal retinal elements of much less acuity and therefore of much less interest than the object of regard.

Construction of Panum's space makes evident another physiologic principle. In order for disparate retinal images to be fused they must be nearly identical in brightness, form, color and direction. If the images are not identical, they cannot be fused despite the fact that they may lie within Panum's fusional space. When nonidentical images fall on corresponding retinal points, as shown with the red and black dots that fall on the respective foveas (Fig. 4.19), "retinal rivalry" occurs. The image from one eye competes with that from the other for conscious regard.

Panum's Fusional Space

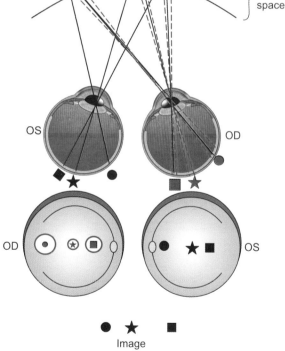

Corresponding Retinal Points

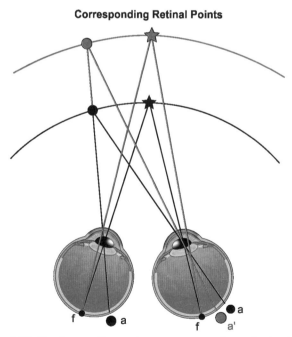

Fig. 4.17: The foveas (f) are always corresponding retinal points, but non-foveal retinal points become corresponding retinal points depending on the distance of the Object of Regard. In this depiction, when the Object of Regard shifts from the black to the red star the corresponding retinal point of "a" in the left eye shifts from "a" to "a′" in the right eye.

Fig. 4.18: There is a zone surrounding any Horopter where slightly disparate objects, striking nearby but not precisely corresponding retinal points can still be fused and seen as a single object. This zone called "Panum's Fusional Space" widens as the distance from the Object of Regard increases. In the retina the zone where non-corresponding retinal points can "fuse" to create a single image is smallest surrounding the fovea and increases as the distance from the fovea increases.

Physiologic Diplopia

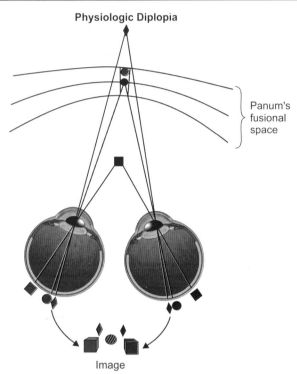

Stereopsis

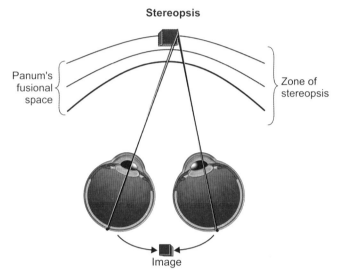

Fig. 4.19: In order to be fused disparate objects must lie within Panum's Fusional Space and must be identical in brightness, form, color and direction. In this depiction the Object of Regard is a black circle. A diamond lies behind Panum's Fusional Space and its image is therefore smaller than the circle. Similarly, because the square lies in front of the black circle its image is larger. In addition, the diamond is closer to Panum's Fusional Space than is the square. Therefore its double image is perceived as being less separated from the circle than the double image of the square. In this depiction the different colors of the images are used to depict the images from the left (red) and right (black) eyes respectively. Also in this depiction a second circle lies within Panum's Fusional Space but is red in color. If the left eye were to fixate on the red circle while the right eye fixated on the black circle retinal rivalry would occur. Even though the red circle lies within Panum's Fusional Space it is not identical to the Object of Regard (different color). The retinal rivalry that would occur is depicted as a black and red striped circle.

Stereopsis

When one looks slightly askance at a cube, the foveas, being only so large, fixate only a small part of the cube. For example, let the part fixated (the object of regard) be the middle of the right edge of the cube. With the eyes fixed on that point, only the image from this point and any other part of the cube that happens to lie on the two-dimensional horopter will fall on corresponding retinal points. However, as can be seen in Figure 4.20, the cube is three dimensional. Every part of the cube that does not lie on the horopter, and therefore whose image falls on noncorresponding retinal elements, is still seen as single because every point on the

Fig. 4.20: The brain is able to perceive that points that lie within Panum's Fusional Space but in front or behind the Horopter are single, and lie in front or behind the object of regard respectively. In this depiction the eyes are focusing on the middle of the right edge of a cube which lies entirely within Panum's Fusional Space. The brain is able to perceive that the cube is a single object. Further, the brain is able to perceive that the back right edge of the cube is in fact in the back and at the right edge of the cube even though the cube lies within Panum's Fusional Space and its image strikes obviously non-corresponding retinal points (the image of the back edge of the cube falls on retinal points nasal to the fovea in both eyes).

cube still lies within Panum's fusional space for the two eyes. Every point that lies on the horopter is perceived as being just as far away as the fixated point on the cube. The multitude of points that lie to one side or the other of the horopter are not just as far away as the fixated point on the cube, and with normal binocular vision the brain is able to perceive this. The brain perceives that any object point whose images fall on noncorresponding retinal points that can still be fused and seen as single (because the point lies within Panum's space) must lie close to the horopter and must be either in front of or behind it.

In Figure 4.20, when the observer fixates the middle of the cube the image of the back edge of the cube falls on retinal elements nasal to the fovea in both eyes. Because the image falls on nasal retina in both eyes, it is obvious that these cannot be corresponding retinal points. Nonetheless, the two retinal points are close enough that they fall within the zone of fusion (the object lies within Panum's space), and the back edge of the cube is seen as one image. The brain is able to discern that if the image lies on fusible retinal elements that are binasally disparate, the object point must lie behind the object of regard (the front edge of the cube). The brain is able to appreciate depth; i.e. it is capable of "stereopsis". In summary, stereopsis results when fusible, but disparate retinal images, arising from object points that lie in front of or behind the horopter but still within Panum's fusional space, stimulate the visual cortex.

In reality, the zone of stereopsis is actually wider than Panum's fusional space, and there is a small zone in front of and behind Panum's space where double images can still be perceived as being farther away or closer than the object of regard.

Tests of Stereopsis

In clinical practice, depth perception is tested using various tests at distant- and near-fixation (Fig. 4.21). Near fixation tests, such as the Titmus (Fig. 4.22), the TNO random dot (Fig. 4.23), and the random dot E (Fig. 4.24), use Polaroid glasses with a card on which slightly disparate objects have been placed. With the first two tests, a series of figures that become more difficult to appreciate stereoscopically allows quantitation of the degree of stereopsis. The smallest stereoscopic target subtends about 20 seconds of arc. A distant stereoscopic test (Fig. 4.25) is also viewed with Polaroid glasses but is projected at 20 feet. The more disparate object subtends 5 minutes of arc (the star), and the smallest 0 minutes of arc (the square). Typically, the observer sees a gradation from the star to the square projected in space, with the star being the closest to the observer.

Monocular Clues in Depth Perception

Although stereopsis may improve the quality of vision, in reality a multitude of monocular clues allow the appreciation of depth. All the monocular clues are the result of experience. Beyond 600 meters, they are the principal clues used to gauge depth. The monocular clues are as follows:

- *Relative size (Fig. 4.26)*: Certain objects are larger than others; e.g. airplanes are larger than birds. If the bird appears as large as or larger than the airplane, it must be closer.

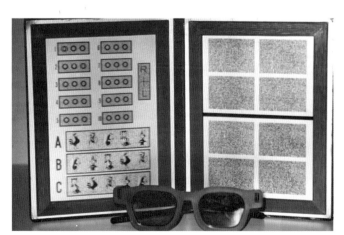

Fig. 4.21: Patient viewing the Titmus test through Polaroid glasses.

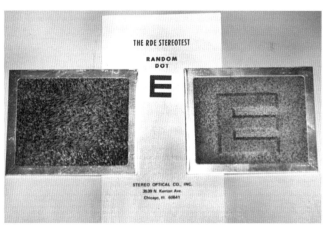

Fig. 4.22: Titmus test of stereopsis.

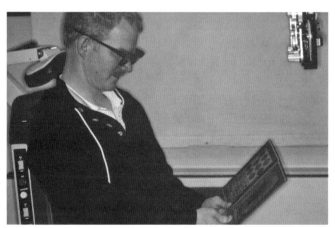

Fig. 4.23: TNO random dot test of stereopsis.

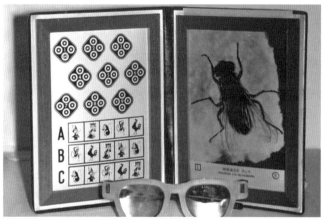

Fig. 4.24: Random dot "E" test of stereopsis.

- *Motion parallax (Fig. 4.27)*: If two objects are viewed directly in line with each other and then the head is rotated to the left while maintaining fixation on these objects, the closer object appears to move a small amount in the direction opposite that of the head rotation, while the farther object appears to make a larger excursion in the same direction as that of the head rotation.

- *Linear perspective (Fig. 4.28)*: Parallel lines appear to converge as they recede from the subject. Railroad tracks appear to approach each other in the distance.
- *Overlay of contours (Fig. 4.29)*: If an object interrupts the contour of a second object, it must lie in front of the second object.
- *Size (Fig. 4.30)*: If an object appears larger than an identical object, it must be closer to the observer.

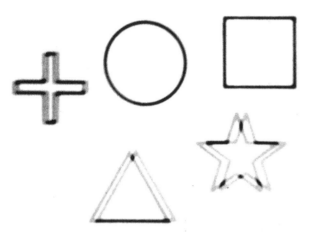

Fig. 4.25: Projected image of a distant stereoscopic test which is viewed with Polaroid glasses at a distance of 20 feet. The star subtends 5 minutes of arc and is perceived as closest and the square is perceived as furthest away.

Monocular Clues to Depth Perception

Relative Size

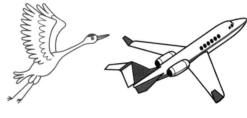

Fig. 4.26: Relative size as a monocular clue to depth perception. If the bird appears as large as an airplane it must be closer than the airplane.

Motion Parallax

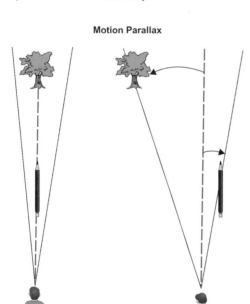

Fig. 4.27: Motion parallax as a monocular clue to depth perception. This phenomenon occurs when an individual rotates her head while viewing two objects that are directly in line with each other. The closer object moves less far than the distant object. In addition the closer object moves in a direction opposite the head turn but the distant object moves in the same direction.

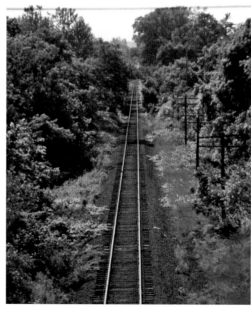

Fig. 4.28: Linear perspective as a monocular clue to depth perception. Parallel lines appear to converge as they recede from the subject.

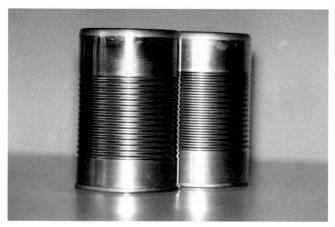

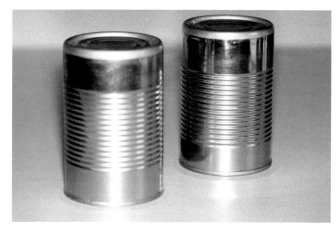

Fig. 4.29: Overlay of contours as a monocular clue to depth perception. An object that interrupts the contour of a second object must lie in front of it.

Fig. 4.30: Size as a monocular clue to depth perception. If an object is larger than an identical object it must be closer.

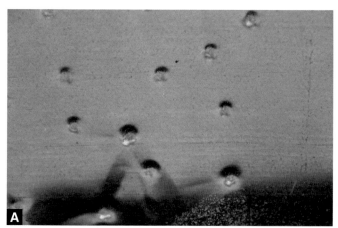

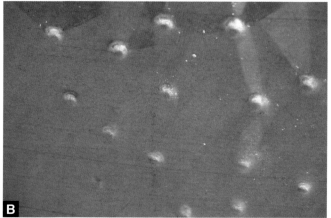

Figs 4.31A and B: Highlights and shadows as a monocular clue to depth perception. (A) When viewing a disruption on vertical surface an indentation is perceived when a shadow is cast above the imperfection and (B) a protrusion is perceived when a shadow is cast below.

- *Highlights and shadows (Figs 4.31A and B)*: Shadows are created by the sunlight above striking objects below. Objects that indent vertical surfaces cast shadows above. Objects that protrude from vertical surfaces cast shadows below.

REFERENCES

1. Parks MM. Single binocular vision. In: Duane TD, Jaeger EA (Eds). Clinical Ophthalmology. Philadelphia: Harper and Row. 1988;1:10-2.

2. Panum PL. Physiologische Untersuchungen über das Sehen mit zwei Augen. Kiel: Schwerssche Buchandlung; 1858.p.52 ff.

BIBLIOGRAPHY

1. Mitchell PR, Parks MM. Single binocular vision. In: Tasman W, Jaeger EA (Eds). Clinical Ophthalmology. Philadelphia: JB Lippincott Co;2013.

2. Scobee RG. The Oculorotatory Muscles. St Louis, Mo: CV Mosby;1947.

3. von Noorden GK, Campos EC. Binocular Vision and Ocular Motility, 6th edition. St Louis, Mo: CV Mosby;2002.

5

Sensory Adaptations to Strabismus

■ SYMPTOMS OF STRABISMUS

If the eyes of a patient who has developed normal binocular vision suddenly become misaligned, two symptoms arise—diplopia and visual confusion.

Diplopia

"Diplopia" (Fig. 5.1) results when the images from a single object fall on retinal points that are too disparate for the

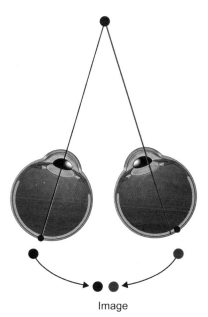

Image

Fig. 5.1: Diplopia. When the eyes of a patient who developed normal binocular vision suddenly become misaligned diplopia results. In this depiction the right eye has turned inward. The Object of Regard still strikes the fovea of the left eye, but now strikes an area nasal to the fovea in the deviating right eye. The image of the object in the deviating right eye will be less clear and to the right of (temporal to) the image from the left eye.

visual system to fuse. Every retinal element has a spatial value that localizes where an object must lie in space when that element is stimulated. In normal binocular vision, there are corresponding retinal points in the two eyes that have the same spatial localization. Upon sudden misalignment of one eye, the image from this eye falls on a retinal element that has a different spatial localization. The two eyes will localize the object to different places, and two images will be seen. The object of regard will still be fixated by one fovea, and this image will always be clearer than the image seen with the noncorresponding, nonfoveal retinal element of the other eye.

Visual Confusion

The partner of diplopia is "visual confusion" (Fig. 5.2). If the image of an object in a misaligned eye falls on a noncorresponding retinal element, some other object must fall on the corresponding element. Confusion arises when the images of two objects that are physically separated in objective space, suddenly fall on corresponding retinal points because the eyes have become misaligned. The visual system localizes these two different objects to the same place in space.

It has been shown experimentally that in persons with normal binocular vision, confusion will not result when different objects are imprinted on the two foveas through the use of occluders and mirrors. It is a physiologic fact that if dissimilar images fall on the two foveas, the image from one or the other fovea is suppressed. Either one fovea is constantly suppressed, or the images on the two foveas compete with each other for conscious regard. This is the basis of "retinal rivalry" and occurs whether the eyes are aligned or not. Confusion is less bothersome than diplopia

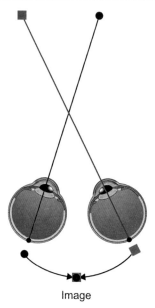

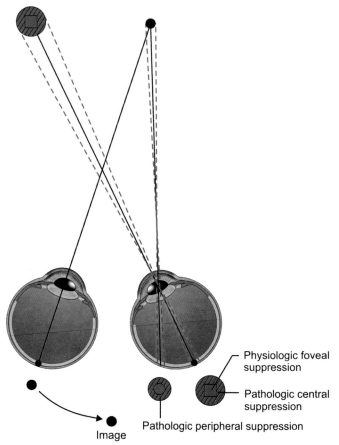

Image

Fig. 5.2: Confusion. When the eyes of a patient who developed normal binocular vision suddenly become misaligned confusion also results. In the same patient depicted in Figure 5.1, the circle is still aligned with the fovea of the left eye, but a square is now aligned with the fovea of the right eye. Even though the circle and the square are physically separated in space they both appear to be originating from the same location in space.

because of "physiologic suppression", but still exists because nonfoveal areas of the retina are not suppressed physiologically.

■ SENSORY ADAPTATIONS

The visual system of a child can adapt, eliminating diplopia and confusion. This adaptation involves the use of suppression and the development of anomalous retinal correspondence.

Suppression

"Suppression" (Fig. 5.3) is the inhibition of the image in one eye from reaching conscious regard. "Physiologic suppression" prevents the appreciation of one of the images when different images fall on the two foveas. In this way, foveal confusion is prevented. Physiologic suppression occurs regardless of the ocular alignment. Pathologic suppression occurs only when the eyes are misaligned. "Pathologic central suppression" inhibits the images that fall near the fovea of the deviating eye from being appreciated, eliminating confusion. "Pathologic peripheral suppression" eliminates diplopia by preventing awareness of the displaced image of the object of regard that arises from a peripheral retinal element of the deviating eye.

Physiologic foveal suppression

Pathologic central suppression

Pathologic peripheral suppression

Image

Fig. 5.3: Suppression. The visual system of a child can adapt to eliminate diplopia and confusion. In this depiction the right eye is deviating inwardly. The brain suppresses the image arising on the fovea of deviating right eye physiologically (physiologic foveal suppression). It also suppresses images that fall near the fovea in the right eye pathologically (pathologic central suppression). This eliminates confusion. In addition, the brain suppresses the image of the Object of Regard that falls on the nasal retina of the deviating right eye to eliminate diplopia (pathologic peripheral suppression).

Suppression can be "monocular" or "alternating", depending on whether one eye becomes dominant. Monocular or unidirectional suppression leads to the development of strabismic amblyopia. Suppression can also be "facultative", meaning that it occurs only when the eyes are misaligned, or "obligatory", meaning that it is present at all times. Furthermore, suppression may be "relative", allowing some visual sensation, or "absolute", inhibiting even the perception of light.

The suppression scotoma is the zone of suppression that occurs when the eyes are misaligned. The majority of patients with strabismus do not suppress the entire retina of the deviating eye. As one approaches the peripheral retina, larger and larger areas of retina in the deviating eye can correspond with areas of the fixating eye. If the visual

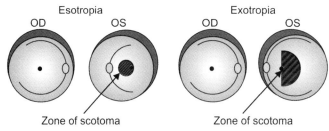

Fig. 5.4: Suppression scotomas. Suppression scotomas in left esotropia and exotropia.

system can fuse these areas of low visual acuity, suppression of these areas need not occur. Furthermore, suppression need not occur for retinal elements whose line of direction is such that objects seen by the deviated eye cannot be seen by the fixating eye. Typically, two suppression scotomas occur in the deviating eye. One lies in the parafoveal area, and the other lies in the peripheral region where the object of regard of the fixating eye is imaged (Fig. 5.3). In very deep suppression the two areas may meld into one, and typically, illustrations of the scotoma in strabismic patients depict this one melded suppression scotoma (Fig. 5.4). Although suppression scotomas can be of any size, the zone that occurs when one eye is turned in (esotropia) is usually roughly circular, encompassing about 5 degrees of nasal retina with the fovea being at the most temporal edge. When one eye is turned out (exotropia) the zone is usually larger and occurs in temporal retina to the hemiretinal line. It is believed that the larger zone in exotropia is due to the variability of the deviation.

Anomalous Retinal Correspondence

In young children, the visual system (probably the visual cortex) can adapt to the misalignment of eyes to retain a crude form of binocularity by shifting the spatial localization of retinal elements in the deviated eye. Retinal elements of the two eyes on which the same images fall develop a common visual direction. Most investigators agree that a suppression scotoma still exists for the fovea of the deviated eye, but for nonfoveal elements new and different correspondence develops; hence "anomalous retinal correspondence" (ARC) (Fig. 5.5). Tests of ARC have been developed based on two different ways to think of ARC. Anomalous retinal correspondence may be viewed as a condition in which the two foveas have different visual directions or as a condition in which an anomalous area of the deviating eye has acquired a common visual direction with the fovea of the fixating eye.

Anomalous retinal correspondence requires a non-changing deviation of sufficient duration for retinocortical

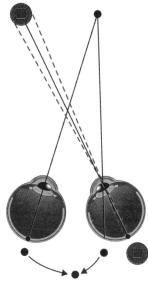

Patient reports

Fig. 5.5: Anomalous retinal correspondence. The visual system of a child with strabismus can also adapt by developing anomalous retinal correspondence. Physiologic foveal and pathologic central suppression still exist to eliminate confusion, but an anomalous area of the retina of the deviating right has acquired a common visual direction with the fovea of the fixating left eye to adapt to (eliminate) diplopia.

relations to become reoriented. Anomalous retinal correspondence may coexist with "normal retinal correspondence" (NRC), with the visual system shifting between the two, depending on the state of ocular alignment. The younger the patient, the more readily ARC develops; it usually cannot develop past middle childhood. Anomalous retinal correspondence is advantageous in eliminating diplopia and tends to stabilize the angle of deviation. It may allow the retention of some depth perception in small deviations.

On realignment of strabismic patients who have ARC, diplopia and visual confusion may return until NRC is re-established. Because the diplopia is in a direction opposite to what might be expected from the position of the eyes, it is called "paradoxical diplopia". Other phenomena such as "monocular diplopia" and "binocular triplopia" may also occur in some patients in whom the ARC is in the process of disintegrating. Until NRC predominates, images in the deviated eye may be localized in two different places as the NRC spatial localization competes with the ARC localization.

■ BIBLIOGRAPHY

1. Crone RA. Diplopia. New York: Elsevier Publishing;1973.
2. Mitchell PR, Parks MM. Sensorial adaptations to strabismus. In: Tasman W, Jaeger EA (Eds). Clinical Ophthalmology. Philadelphia: JB Lippincott;2013.

6

Tests of the Sensory Status

■ THE WORTH'S FOUR DOT TEST

The "Worth's four dot test" determines whether suppression of one eye is occurring under binocular conditions. The patient looks through a pair of red and green glasses at a target consisting of four illuminated colored dots (Figs 6.1A and B). The dots are arranged as a diamond. The two horizontal dots are green, the top vertical dot is red and the bottom vertical dot is white. The patient sees the green dots with the eye looking through the green lens, and the red dot with the other eye. With normal binocular vision, the white dot is alternately seen as a mixture of red or green as a result of retinal rivalry (Fig. 6.2).

In a patient with strabismus different responses can occur, depending on the size of the suppression scotoma and the distance of the target (Figs 6.3A and B). When the test is conducted at distant fixation, a small central field of the retina is stimulated; when the target is brought closer to the patient a larger and more peripheral field is stimulated. If the suppression scotoma is small, the image of the target may fall completely within the scotoma at distant fixation but outside the scotoma at near fixation. While a suppression response may occur at a distance, at near fixation the patient may report seeing either four or five dots. If a patient with obviously misaligned eyes reports a normal response (four dots), the visual direction of the retinal elements of the misaligned eye must have been reoriented, and the patient has anomalous retinal correspondence (ARC). If the patient reports seeing five dots (diplopia response), normal retinal correspondence (NRC) must prevail.

■ THE RED GLASS TEST

The "red glass test" utilizes a red filter placed before the fixating eye while the patient fixates a bright light

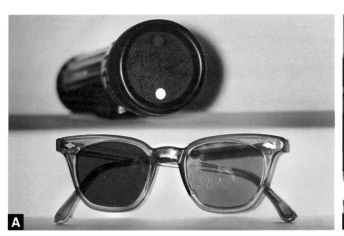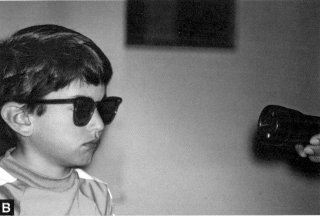

Figs 6.1A and B: Worth's four dot test: (A) Flashlight and glasses used; (B) Test being performed.

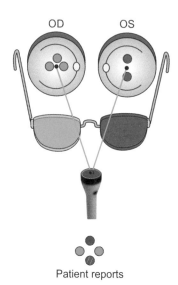

Fig. 6.2: Report of a patient with normal binocular vision on Worth's four dot test.

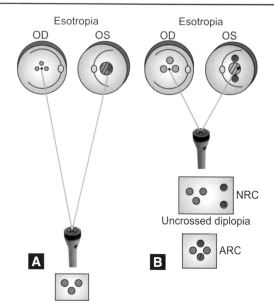

Figs 6.3A and B: Worth four dot test results on a patient with esotropia at distant (A) and near (B) fixation. A: At distant fixation a patient with a left esotropia and a suppression scotoma reports only seeing the image from the fixating right eye. B: As the flashlight is brought closer to the eye the image in the deviating eye falls outside the suppression scotoma and the patient now reports seeing four or five dots. If the patient reports seeing five dots they have maintained normal retinal correspondence (NRC). If the patient reports seeing only four dots anomalous retinal correspondence (ARC) has developed.

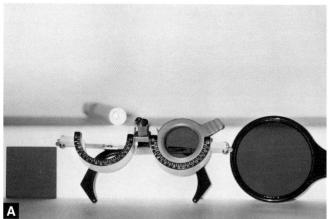

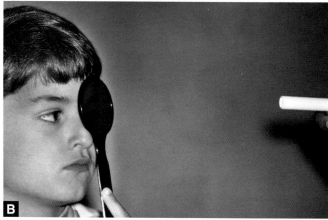

Figs 6.4A and B: The red glass test: (A) Different red lenses that can be used including a simple square lens, a red lens that can be placed in a trial frame and a red lens occluder. (B) Red glass test being performed.

(Figs 6.4A and B). When a patient with misaligned eyes does not complain of diplopia, the red glass test is used to determine whether he or she is suppressing the second image or has developed ARC. If the second image has not been consciously appreciated, this test will draw the patient's attention to it by stimulating the retina of the deviated eye with a bright white light that is contrasted with the less intense red light stimulating the fovea of the fixating eye.

In the patient with NRC, if the white light falls outside the suppression scotoma, two images are seen (Fig. 6.5A). In the patient with esotropia, these images are uncrossed ("homonymous diplopia") because the image

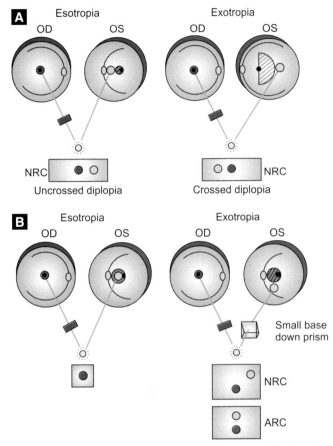

Figs 6.5A and B: Results of the red glass test: (A) A patient with a left esotropia, small suppression scotoma and normal retinal correspondence (NRC) will report uncrossed diplopia with the image from the inward deviating left eye being displaced temporally. A patient with left exotropia and NRC will report crossed diplopia with the image from the outward deviating left eye being displaced nasally. (B) A patient with left esotropia and a large and deep suppression scotoma will report only seeing the image from the fixating eye in front of which a red lens has been placed (a single red light). An additional test is used to determine if she has maintained NRC or has developed anomalous retinal correspondence (ARC). A small base down prism is introduced in front of the deviating eye. If she reports now also seeing a white light which is temporally and upwardly displaced from the red light she has maintained NRC. If the white light is directly on top of the red light she has developed ARC.

in the deviated eye falls on nasal retina and is projected temporally in space (to the same side as the deviated eye). In the patient with exotropia and NRC, the images are crossed ("heteronymous diplopia") because in this case the light falls on temporal retina and is projected nasally.

If the white light falls within a deep suppression scotoma (Fig. 6.5B), the patient may report seeing only the red light. Because a diplopia response is not given, it

is not known whether ARC or NRC exists. By placing a small base-down prism in front of the deviating eye, one can vertically displace the image falling on this eye. In the patient with NRC, a diplopia response is given with the white light above the red light and to the same side as the deviating eye (uncrossed-esotropia) or opposite side (crossed-exotropia). If the patient reports that the two dots are separated vertically but not horizontally, ARC must exist because the two retinas having the same visual direction except for the vertical displacement of the image induced by the prism in front of the deviating eye.

The red glass test can also be used to map out the size of the suppression scotoma by displacing the image in the deviating eye with larger and larger prisms until a white light is appreciated. Another use of this test is to measure the gaze position of greatest misalignment in incomitant strabismus by having the patient indicate the distance between the diplopic images as his or her eyes are rotated through the diagnostic positions of gaze.

■ THE AFTERIMAGE TEST

The "afterimage test" differs from other tests of sensory status in several important respects. Along with examination with the major amblyoscope, it is the only test in which each eye is stimulated separately to specifically label and determine the visual direction of the fovea of each eye. Other tests are done binocularly, during which the nondominant eye is misaligned and is not directed at the object of regard. The afterimage test is done monocularly, and the nondominant eye, when stimulated, is looking at the object of regard. Instead of determining, in the nondominant eye, where the image lies with regard to the fovea, this test elicits where the fovea is directed with regard to the retinal element in the nondominant eye whose spatial orientation is straight ahead. This test labels the foveas of each eye. Of all the sensory tests, the afterimage test is the most dissociative. An ARC response with this test indicates that the ARC is deep-seated.

The test is performed by using any tubular light source that can be flashed at a patient and can be pivoted and oriented in either a horizontal or a vertical direction. The patient's gaze is directed to an occluding band in the middle of the filament (Figs 6.6A and B). First, the fovea of the eye with better acuity is labeled, with the filament directed horizontally for 20 seconds in a darkened room while the other eye is occluded. The occluder is then

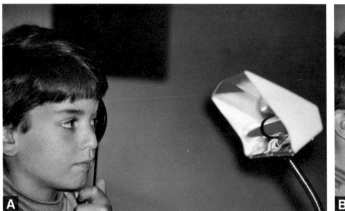

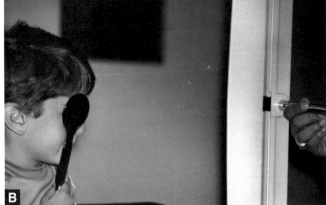

Figs 6.6A and B: Performance of the afterimage test: (A) A tubular light source with an occluding central band is shown horizontally in front of the eye with the better acuity. (B) The light source is then rotated vertically (90 degrees) and shown to the opposite eye. For both eyes the patient is asked to fixate on the occluding central band of the tubular light source.

switched to the first eye, and the fovea of the second eye is labeled while the filament is directed vertically. The occluder and light are removed, and the patient is asked to indicate the direction of the afterimages (Figs 6.7A and B). In the patient with NRC, the visual direction of the foveas of both eyes is toward the object of regard. If the gaps in the center of the afterimage are superimposed, the foveas must have the same visual direction regardless of the alignment of the eyes. In the patient with ARC, some other retinal element of the deviated eye (f′) has the same visual direction as the fovea of the dominant eye under binocular conditions; the fovea (f) of the deviated eye has a different spatial localization. In the patient with esotropia (Fig. 6.7A) and ARC the fovea of the nondominant eye (f) is temporal to the retinal element (f′), which corresponds to the fovea of the dominant eye. The vertical afterimage [or spatial location of the fovea (f) of the nondominant eye] is therefore displaced nasally (or crossed). In the patient with exotropia (Fig. 6.7B) and ARC the fovea (f) is nasal to the retinal element (f′), which corresponds to the fovea of the dominant eye and the vertical afterimage is displaced temporally (uncrossed).

The afterimage test is of limited use in the individual with eccentric fixation, in whom a nonfoveal area of the deviated eye will be labeled, preventing an assessment of the visual direction of the fovea. Patients who can readily switch from NRC to ARC, as is seen in some patients with an intermittent deviation, may report seeing the afterimages form a cross when the eyes are aligned but separate when the eyes are deviated. This change is not due to movement of the nondominant eye but to a switch from NRC to ARC when the nondominant eye is allowed to deviate.

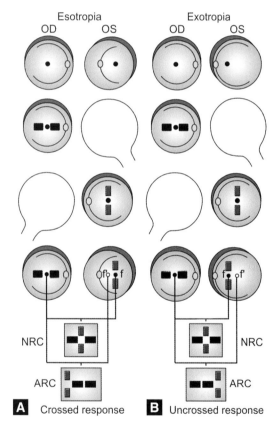

Figs 6.7A and B: The afterimage test in patients with left esotropia (A) and left exotropia (B). In each case fovea of the fixating right eye is labeled first with the filament directed horizontally. The occluder is then switched and the deviating left eye is labeled with the filament directed vertically. Patients with normal retinal correspondence (NRC) will report that the gaps in the center of the afterimages are superimposed. In patients with anomalous retinal correspondence (ARC) some other retinal area of the deviating eye (f′) has the same visual direction as the fovea of the dominant eye (f). The patient with esotropia and ARC reports that vertical afterimage is nasally displaced; the patient with exotropia and NRC reports it to be temporally displaced.

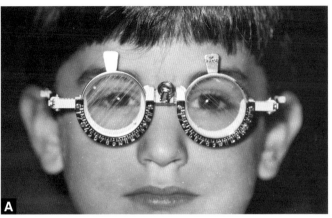 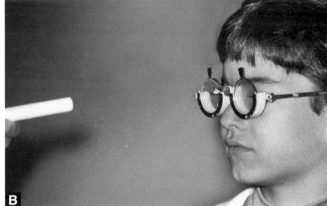

Figs 6.8A and B: Bagolini's striated glass test: (A) Bagolini lenses placed in opposite directions (45° and 135°) in a trial frame; (B) Bagolini's striated glass test being performed.

THE BAGOLINI'S STRIATED GLASS TEST

The "Bagolini's striated glass test" uses pieces of glass without any refracting power on which nearly imperceptible parallel striations have been made. The environment is minimally distorted when the patient looks through a Bagolini lens, and therefore, this test least dissociates the eyes. Because of this minimal dissociative effect, the Bagolini test is more sensitive in detecting a tenuous ARC. The same patient who tests as having NRC with the very dissociative afterimage test may demonstrate ARC with the Bagolini test.

The test is performed by placing one lens with the striations at 45° in front of the right eye and a second lens with the striations at 135° in front of the left eye. The patient fixates a light source, and the striations act as a Maddox rod (see Fig. 7.34) to image a streak of light on the retina at 90° to the striations on the glass (Figs 6.8A and B). The patient whose eyes are aligned (orthophoria) reports seeing the lines cross with the point light source in the center. The image from the right eye is oriented at 45° (the same as the striations on the glass in front of this eye), and the image from the left eye is oriented at 135° (Fig. 6.9).

If a patient with a manifest ocular deviation reports seeing only one light source, suppression is present. In the patient with strabismus and NRC, the image of the light source falls on a noncorresponding retinal element, and two lights should be seen unless this area of the retina is being suppressed. The images of the induced streaks of light are used to determine whether the patient who sees only one light source has NRC and suppression or ARC and suppression. In the patient with esotropia, the image on the retina is nasally displaced, and the esotropic patient with

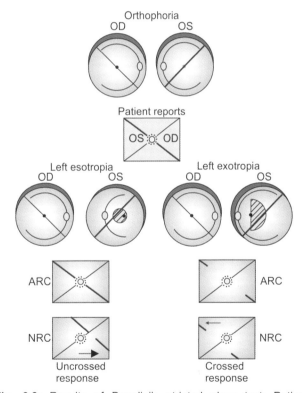

Fig. 6.9: Results of Bagolini's striated glass test: Patients with orthophoria report seeing a single light with lines crossing at 45° and 135° through the center of the light. Patients with a suppression scotoma and anomalous retinal correspondence (ARC) will also report seeing a single light with the lines crossing at 45° and 135° through the center of the light but there is a gap in the line image from the deviating eye. This gap will be larger in exotropic patients. Patients with a suppression scotoma and normal retinal correspondence (NRC) will report that the line image from the deviating eye does not cross through the light. In esotropic patients with NRC the line will be temporally displaced (uncrossed) and in exotropic patients with NRC it will be nasally displaced (crossed).

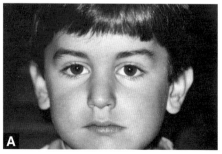 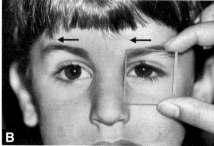 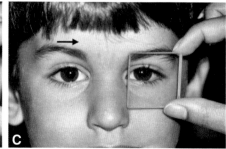

Figs 6.10A to C: The four diopter base-out prism test being performed on a child with bifoveal fixation. Introduction of a base-out four diopter prism in front of the left eye of this patient initially causes both eyes move to the right followed by a slow inward movement of just the right eye.

NRC reports the streak as being displaced temporally in space. In the patient with exotropia, the image on the retina is temporally displaced, and the patient with exotropia and NRC reports the streak as being nasally displaced. In the patient with ARC the streaks still cross at the light source.

It is also noted that the streak from the deviated eye may be interrupted. This occurs when the image in the deviated eye falls on an area of the retina being suppressed. If the entire retina is suppressed, only the streak from the fixating eye is appreciated. Because the suppression scotoma in exotropia is usually larger than the scotoma in esotropia, the interruption of t1he streak in exotropia is usually longer.

THE FOUR DIOPTER BASE-OUT PRISM TEST

The "four diopter base-out prism test" is used to detect a small central suppression scotoma in patients with microstrabismus or the monofixation syndrome. In patients with bifoveal fixation, the introduction of a small base-out prism in front of one eye brings about a binocular refixation movement followed by a monocular fusional movement in the opposite eye (Figs 6.10A to C and 6.11A).

On immediate introduction of a base-out prism in front of one eye the image in this eye is displaced temporally. If the patient was previously fixating with both foveas, a reflex nasal refixation movement of this eye occurs. Because of Hering's law, the fellow eye simultaneously moves temporally. However, at this point the image is temporally displaced in the fellow eye. To maintain bifixation, a slow monocular fusional movement of the second eye will occur until bifixation is again achieved (Fig. 6.11A).

If the patient is suppressing one fovea, the complete biphasic response does not occur. What does occur depends on whether the prism is introduced in front of the

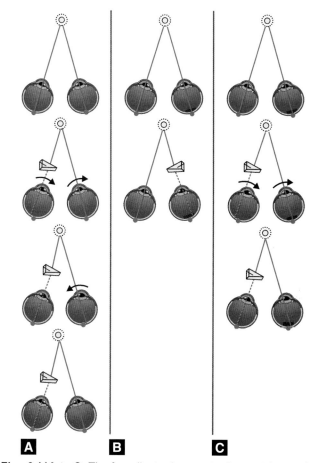

Figs 6.11A to C: The four diopter base-out prism test in a patient with bifoveal fixation (A), and a patient with right esotropia with foveal suppression (B and C). In B the prism is introduced in front of the deviating right eye with foveal suppression. In C the prism is introduced in front of the fixating left eye.

fixating eye or the eye with the suppression scotoma. If the prism is brought in front of the eye with the suppression scotoma (Fig. 6.11B), the image is moved from one area of nonappreciated (scotomatous) retina to another.

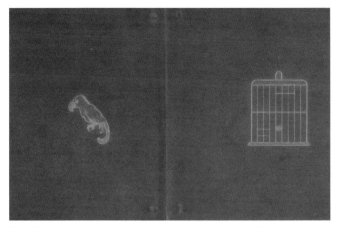

Fig. 6.12: Separate test objects presented to the foveas of each eye by the major amblyoscope. In this example a bird is presented to the right eye and a cage to the left eye.

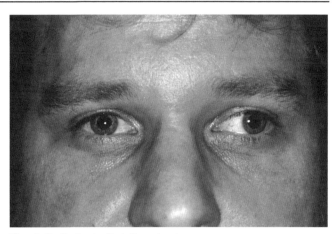

Fig. 6.13: Patient with left exotropia.

No movement of either eye occurs. If the prism is introduced in front of the fixating eye (Fig. 6.11C), this eye demonstrates the fixational reflex and turns in, and the fellow eye simultaneously turns out according to Hering's law. However, the second fusional movement of the opposite eye does not occur, as the shift of the image in the second eye is not appreciated.

■ THE MAJOR AMBLYOSCOPE

The "major amblyoscope" (synoptophore, troposcope) is useful in determining the angle of strabismus, the degree and range of fusion, and the sensory status of the eyes. It functions as a "haploscopic test", in which separate test objects are presented to each fovea, such as a bird and a cage (Fig. 6.12), and the patient is eventually asked to superimpose them (i.e. place the bird inside the cage). In the patient with strabismus (Fig. 6.13) each eye sees only one of the targets through a tube that can be adjusted horizontally and vertically as well as cyclorotationally (Fig. 6.14). The amounts of all of these rotations can be read from graduated scales. The targets are placed in the focal planes of high-plus lenses (+ 6.00) to prevent accommodation from affecting the deviation.

To test the sensory status of the patient with strabismus, both arms of the amblyoscope are moved by the examiner while presenting the separate targets alternately to the two eyes until no fixation movements of the eyes occur. When the fixation movements cease, it means that the targets are aligned with their respective foveas. The target for the right

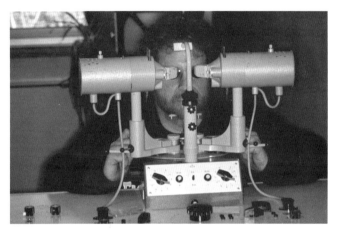

Fig. 6.14: Patient in Figure 6.13 being tested on the major amblyoscope. Initially separate test objects are presented to each fovea and the tubes of the amblyoscope are adjusted horizontally, vertically and cyclorotationally to determine the "objective angle of deviation".

eye is directed at the right fovea, and the target for the left eye is directed at the left fovea, so that when either eye is shown its target, it does not have to move to centrally fixate it. This establishes the "objective angle" of the deviation as indicated on the scale of the instrument (Fig. 6.15). As long as the patient does not have eccentric fixation, he or she fixates with the fovea of each eye under monocular conditions, and the targets are directed to the foveas of both eyes. Both targets are then simultaneously illuminated and the patient is asked what he or she sees. If the patient sees the targets superimposed, his or her foveas have the same visual direction, and NRC is present (Fig. 6.16).

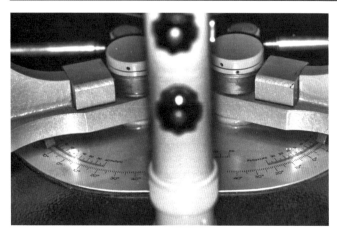

Fig. 6.15: The objective angle of deviation for the patient in Figure 6.13 is read from the scales on the instrument.

If after aligning the targets with the foveas of each eye the patient reports that the targets are separated when viewed simultaneously, under binocular conditions the fovea of the patient's deviating eye must have a visual direction different than that of the fovea of the dominant eye; ARC must be present.

The patient with ARC (whose "subjective angle" of deviation does not equal his or her objective angle of deviation) is then asked to move the arms of the amblyoscope to superimpose the images. By moving the arms of the amblyoscope, the target in the deviating eye is displaced away from the fovea and toward the retinal element in the deviating eye, which corresponds to the fovea of the dominant eye. The true angle of deviation that had been determined under monocular conditions is reduced under binocular conditions through the patient's use of ARC. This is reflected in the reduced scale reading on the amblyoscope when the patient is allowed to use both eyes together. If the arms are set to zero, as if no deviation were present (Fig. 6.17), this indicates complete reorientation of the patient's deviated retina, so that when the eyes are allowed to assume their resting deviated state (see Fig. 6.13) there is no subjective misalignment of the images despite an obvious objective misalignment of the eyes. This is called "harmonious ARC" (Fig. 6.18). If the arms are set somewhere in between so that the target in the deviating eye does not fall on the fovea but also does not fall on the expected peripheral retinal element corresponding to the degree of misalignment of the eye, the reorientation of retinal elements is not precisely in line with the objective deviation.

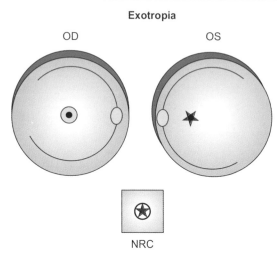

Fig. 6.16: The images seen through the major amblyoscope when presented simultaneously to a patient with normal retinal correspondence. Note that images (in this example a circle directed to the fovea of the right eye and a star directed to the fovea of the left eye) appear to the patient to be superimposed. A patient with anomalous retinal correspondence would report that the images are separated.

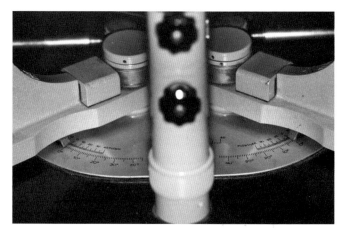

Fig. 6.17: After establishing the objective angle of deviation for the patient in Figure 6.13, the patient was allowed to view the objects simultaneously. This patient reported that the targets were separated (indicating anomalous retinal correspondence) and he was asked to move the arms of the amblyoscope to superimpose the images. Upon superimposing the images the scales of the amblyoscope were re-read establishing his "subjective angle of deviation". This patient reduced the scale reading of the amblyoscope to zero.

The arms of the amblyoscope will be set between zero and the objective angle, and the patient is said to have "unharmonious ARC".

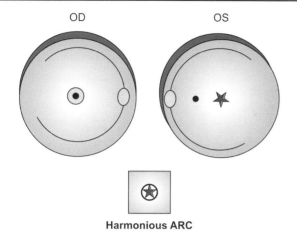

OD   OS

Harmonious ARC

Fig. 6.18: Because the patient in Figure 6.13 with an apparent exotropia reset the arms of the amblyoscope to zero (as if no deviation were present) he has complete or harmonious ARC. He sees the circle and the star as aligned despite the star being projected onto a nonfoveal area of his left retina.

Whether unharmonious ARC truly exists has been questioned. The sensation of nearness brought on by the target's being close to the eyes may cause the eyes to converge, artificially changing the subjective angle of the deviation. However, in other instances, such as the monofixation syndrome, extramacular fusion can decrease the angle of deviation measured under binocular conditions.

■ BIBLIOGRAPHY

1. Bagolini B. Anomalous correspondence: definition and diagnostic methods. Doc Ophthalmol. 1967;23:346.
2. Lang J. Evaluation in small angle strabismus or microtropia. In: Arruga A (Ed). International Strabismus Symposium. Basel and New York: S Karger AG;1968.
3. von Noorden GK, Campos EC. Binocular vision and ocular motility. 6th edition. St Louis, MO: CV Mosby;2002.

7

Introduction to Strabismus

DEFINITIONS

Individuals with "orthophoria" or "straight eyes" simultaneously direct both eyes at the object of regard even when a cover is placed in front of one eye. "Heterophoria" is the state in which sensory fusion keeps an ocular deviation latent, as demonstrated in the patient in Figures 7.1A and B whose eye turns out when an occluder is placed in front of one eye. A looser, albeit incorrect, use of the term orthophoria allows a small heterophoria (approximately half diopter of hyperphoria, 1–2 diopters of esophoria, or 1–4 diopters of exophoria) to be present when fusion is suspended. "Heterotropia" is used to indicate that an ocular deviation is present at all times.

"Strabismus" (Greek, "to squint or look obliquely at") is another general term meaning dissociated or misaligned eyes. Heterophoria is considered latent strabismus, and heterotropia is considered manifest strabismus; the two suffixes "-phoria" and "-tropia" distinguish latent from manifest deviations. Different prefixes describe the direction the deviated eye is turned. "Esotropia" (Fig. 7.2) means that the visual axis of the deviated eye is directed inward. "Exotropia" (Fig. 7.3) describes a divergent position of the deviated eye. "Hypertropia" (Fig. 7.4) means that the deviated eye is turned upward, and "hypotropia" (Fig. 7.5) downward. Esophoria, exophoria, hyperphoria and hypophoria describe the respective latent counterparts. Strabismus is categorized with respect to the nonfixating eye. This is useful in identifying the deviating eye in vertical strabismus. A left hypotropia appropriately identifies the deviating eye in Figure 7.5 as opposed to describing this patient as having a right hypertropia.

CLASSIFICATION SCHEMES

In addition to classifying strabismus according to fusional status and direction of deviation, strabismus is also classified according to age of onset, fixation preference,

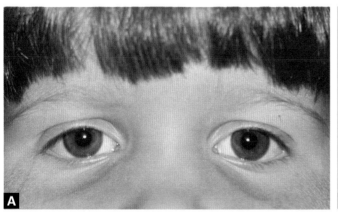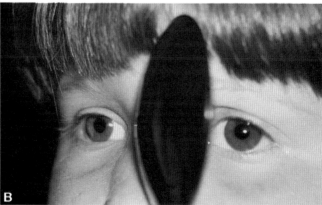

Figs 7.1A and B: Heterophoria: (A) With neither eye occluded sensory fusion keeps this child's ocular deviation latent; (B) Upon occlusion of one eye, the occluded eye deviates (in this child it turns outward).

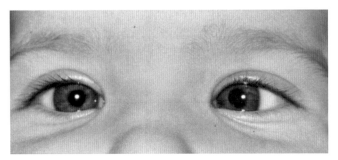

Fig. 7.2: Left esotropia.

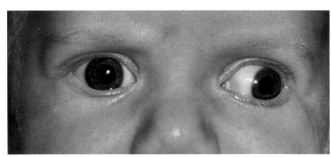

Fig. 7.3: Left exotropia.

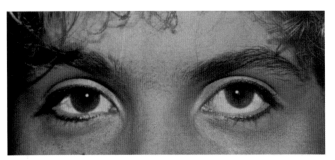

Fig. 7.4: Left hypertropia.
Courtesy: Joseph H Calhoun.

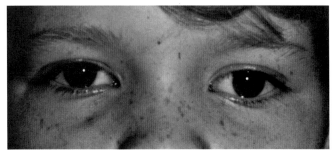

Fig. 7.5: Left hypotropia.
Courtesy: Donelson R Manley.

Table 7.1: Classification parameters of strabismus	
Fusional status	Phoria: Latent Tropis: Manifest Intermittent: Occasionally manifest
Direction of deviation	Horizontal: Esodeviation, exodeviation Vertical: Hyperdeviation, hypodeviation Torsional: Incyclodeviation, excyclodeviation
Age of onset	Congenital: Prior to 6 months of age Acquired: After 6 months of age
Fixation preference	Monocular: Definite preference for one eye Alternating: No ocular preference
Variation with gaze position	Comitant: Does not vary Incomitant: Varies with direction of gaze
Distant-and near-fixation relationship	Normal AC/A: Same deviation at distant and near fixation High AC/A: Excessive convergence with accommodation Low AC/A: Deficient convergence with accommodation

variation of the deviation with gaze position, and the distant- and near-fixation relationship (Table 7.1).

"Congenital" describes any strabismus present by 6 months of age regardless of whether it was noted at birth. A better term may be "infantile". All other deviations are considered "acquired". If a fixation preference exists such that one eye always deviates under binocular conditions, the term "monocular" is used (Figs 7.6A to C). Note in this patient that her nondominant left eye picks up fixation when her dominant right eye is occluded. As soon as the occluder is removed, fixation reverts to her right eye. In the patient with monocular strabismus, the nondominant eye is often amblyopic. The opposing situation, in which fixation spontaneously alternates or can be switched by occluding the fixating eye, is termed "alternate" strabismus (Figs 7.7A to C).

If the deviation varies depending on the gaze position, the term "incomitant" is used. A "comitant" deviation does not vary regardless of the position of the eyes. Four major categories of incomitance exist: restrictive, innervational, muscular and oblique dysfunction (Table 7.2).

A final classification considers the relationship of accommodation to the deviation. Accommodation is linked to convergence (discussed later in this chapter). If excessive convergence accompanies accommodation, the accommodative convergence to accommodation "(AC/A)" ratio is said to be "high". Such a ratio occurs especially with accommodative esotropia. The opposite condition, in which convergence is subnormal for accommodation, is called a "low AC/A" ratio. An example is convergence insufficiency.

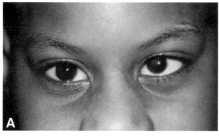
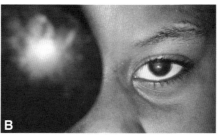
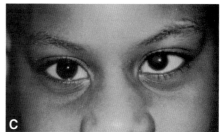

Figs 7.6A to C: Monocular strabismus: (A) This child is fixating with her right eye and her left eye is turned inward; (B) Upon occlusion of her right eye she picks up fixation with her left eye; (C) As soon as the occluder is removed she regains fixation with her right eye and her left eye again deviates. Her right eye is dominant.

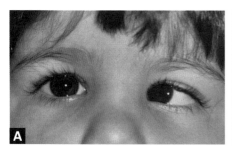
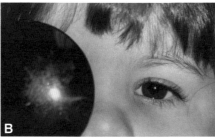
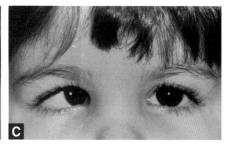

Figs 7.7A to C: Alternating strabismus: (A) This child is fixating with her right eye and her left eye is turned inward; (B) Upon occlusion of her right eye she picks up fixation with her left eye; (C) Upon removal of the occluder she maintains fixation with her left eye. Neither eye is dominant.

Table 7.2: Causes of incomitant strabismus
Restrictive Incomitant Strabismus
Inflammation: Cellulitis, pseudotumor, thyroid ophthalmopathy, orbital tumor
Trauma: Orbital fracture, orbital surgery, previous strabismus surgery
Innervational Incomitant Strabismus
Congenital: Congenital cranial nerve dysfunction (e.g. Duane's syndrome)
Cranial nerve palsy: Trauma, aneurysm, diabetes, tumor, demyelination, inflammation, increased intracranial pressure, temporal arteritis
Internuclear lesion: Demyelination, vascular accident, tumor
Neuromuscular junction: Myasthenia gravis
Degenerative: Chronic progressive external ophthalmoplegia
Muscular
Myositis, thyroid ophthalmopathy, musculofascial syndromes (e.g. Brown's syndrome), agenesis of extraocular muscle
Oblique Muscle Dysfunction

In measuring deviations at near fixation, the influence of accommodation must be controlled by having the patient fixate an accommodative target at a near distance, such as small letters or a detailed picture. A penlight is not an accommodative target. A large deviation at a near fixation may be entirely missed if the patient fixates on a light source as opposed to fixating on a descriptive accommodative target (Figs 7.8A and B).

Measurement of the AC/A Ratio

Normally, the eye converges 3–6 prism diopters (Δ) per diopter (D) of accommodation, depending on the method used to measure this parameter. Three methods exist for determining the AC/A ratio (Table 7.3). They are the distant versus near deviation method, the heterophoria method, and the lens gradient method.

Distant Versus Near Deviation

The patient with a "normal AC/A" ratio has a similar alignment at near and distant fixation. If the patient is more esotropic, or less exotropic when fixating at a near distance, an excessive amount of convergence accompanies accommodation ("high AC/A"). If the patient is more exotropic, or less esotropic when fixating at a near distance, deficient accommodative convergence accompanies accommodation.

The AC/A ratio is frequently clinically evaluated by simply comparing the amount of deviation at near fixation (1/3 meter) with the deviation at a distant fixation (6 meters).

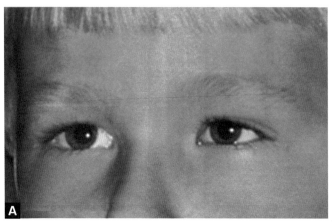 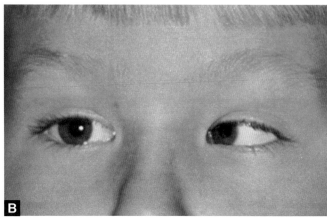

Figs 7.8A and B: The influence of accommodation on ocular deviations at near fixation. (A) No ocular deviation is apparent when this child viewed a non-accommodating target (a penlight); (B) Upon viewing an accommodating target a large esodeviation becomes manifest.

Table 7.3: The determination of the AC/A ratio		
Classification	*Distant Fixation*	*Near Fixation*
Normal AC/A	Orthophoria	Orthophoria
	ET*	Same ET
	XT*	Same XT
High AC/A	Orthophoria	ET
	ET	Greater ET
	XT	Less XT or orthophoria
Low AC/A	Orthophoria	XT
	ET	Less ET or orthophoria
	XT	Greater XT

Methods

Distant versus Near deviation

Compare deviation at distant (6 meters) and near (1/3 meter) fixation. High AC/A = an esotropic shift of 10-prism diopters or more

Heterophoria method

$$AC/A = IPD + \frac{(\Delta_{near} - \Delta_{distance})}{D_{near}}$$

where: IPD = interpupillary distance in centimeters
Δ_{near} = near deviation in prism diopters
$\Delta_{distance}$ = distant deviation in prism diopters
D_{near} = fixation distance at near in diopters
D = 1/fixation distance (in meters)

Lens gradient method

$$AC/A = \frac{\Delta_{original} - \Delta_{lens}}{D}$$

where: $\Delta_{original}$ = the original deviation in prism diopters
Δ_{lens} = the deviation in prism diopters looking through an ophthalmic lens
D = the dioptric power of the lens

*ET: Esotropia; XT: Exotropia

Similar prism and cover measurements at the two fixations indicates a normal AC/A ratio. An esodeviation that is greater by 10 prism diopters or more at near fixation is often considered abnormally high. Although clinically useful, this 10-prism diopter difference is a rough estimation of abnormality that does not take into account the interpupillary distance.

The Heterophoria Method

The heterophoria method takes into account the interpupillary distance in comparing the far and near deviations. The AC/A ratio is determined using the equation:

$$AC/A = IPD + \frac{(\Delta_{near} - \Delta_{distance})}{D_{near}}$$

where: IPD = interpupillary distance in centimeters (cm)
Δ_{near} = near deviation in prism diopters (Δ)
$\Delta_{distance}$ = distance deviation in prism diopters (Δ)
D_{near} = near fixation distance given in terms of diopters
D = 1/fixation distance (in meters)

By convention, esodeviations are positive (+), and exodeviations are negative (–).
If IPD = 5.0 cm, $\Delta_{near} = 30^\Delta$ ET; Δ distance = 20^Δ ET, and the fixation distance at near = 1/3 meter:

AC/A = 5.0 + (30 – 20)/3
AC/A = 8.33 Δ/D

If IPD = 6.0 cm, $\Delta_{near} = 16^\Delta$ XT; $\Delta_{distance} = 0^\Delta$, and the fixation distance at near is 1/4 meter:

AC/A = 6.0 + (–16 – 0)/4
AC/A = 2.0 Δ/D

The Lens Gradient Method

The lens gradient method may give the truest estimate of the AC/A ratio because the determination is made with the fixation distance being held constant, eliminating the effect of proximal convergence. Ocular deviations are measured with the prism and cover test at a fixed fixation distance, using ophthalmic lenses to stimulate or relax accommodation. Plus lenses relax and minus lenses stimulate accommodation. It is assumed that within a certain range the accommodative convergence response to varying accommodative needs is linear. The AC/A ratio is determined using the equation:

$$AC/A \frac{\Delta_{\text{original}} - \Delta_{\text{lens}}}{D}$$

where: Δ_{original} = the original deviation in prism diopters

Δ_{lens} = the deviation in prism diopters looking through an ophthalmic lens

D = the dioptic power of the lens

Again, esodeviations are positive, and exodeviations are negative.

If the original deviation was 30^Δ ET and became 12^Δ ET looking through a + 3.00 lens:

$$AC/A = (30 - 12)/3$$
$$AC/A = 6.0 \ \Delta/D$$

If the original deviation was 20^Δ XT and became 0^Δ looking through a – 2.00 lens:

$$AC/A = (-20 - 0)/-2$$
$$AC/A = 10 \ \Delta/D$$

To ensure accuracy in using the gradient method, more than one determination should be made to be sure that the measurements have been made under conditions in which the AC/A ratio is linear.

■ UNITS OF MEASURE AND INSTRUMENTS USED TO QUANTITATE ALIGNMENT

Degrees of Deviation and Prism Diopters

Some tests (e.g. Hirschberg's test) measure an ocular deviation in degrees, whereas most other tests measure a deviation in prism diopters. A "degree" is an angular measure equal in magnitude to the angle that subtends 1/360 of the circumference of a circle. One "prism diopter" is a 1-cm deflection of a light ray measured at 100 cm from the prism. Light is always deflected toward the base of the prism (Fig. 7.9).

The relationship between degrees of deviation and prism diopters is a trigonometric one in which 1 prism diopter equals 100 times the tangent of the angle in degrees. For less than 100 prism diopters, which encompasses most uses in ophthalmology, 1° is approximately equal to 2 prism diopters. However, the number of prism diopters per degree increases exponentially beyond 100 prism diopters (45°) (Fig. 7.10).

Ophthalmic Prisms

Two different types of ophthalmic prisms exist. A 40 prism-diopter glass prism is shown on the left, and a 40 prism-diopter plastic prism is shown on the right in Figure 7.12.

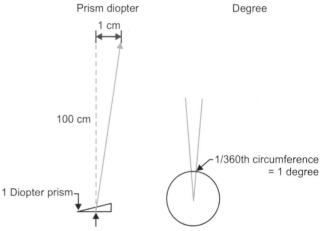

Prism Diopters Versus Degrees

Fig. 7.9: Difference between a prism diopter and a degree. A one diopter prism deflects a ray of light 1 cm at 100 cm from the prism. One degree is an angular measure equal to the angle that subtends 1/360th of the perimeter of a circle.

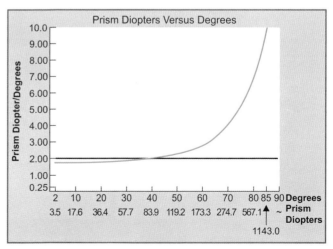

Fig. 7.10: Despite its trigonometric relationship one degree is approximately equal to 2 prism diopters for most of the prisms used in ophthalmology (prisms smaller than 100 prism diopters).

"Glass prisms" are calibrated according to "Prentice's position", which requires that light rays strike one of the surfaces of the prism perpendicularly. However, "plastic prisms" are calibrated according to the "angle of minimal deviation", which requires equal bending of the light rays at the two surfaces (Fig. 7.11).

Errors in holding prisms may result in errors in the measured deviation, as shown for a glass prism placed in the frontal plane (Fig. 7.13). The correct way to hold a glass prism is with the rear surface at 90° to the deviated eye's visual axis (Fig. 7.14). Plastic prisms should be held with the rear surface in the frontal plane (Fig. 7.15).

Ophthalmic Prisms

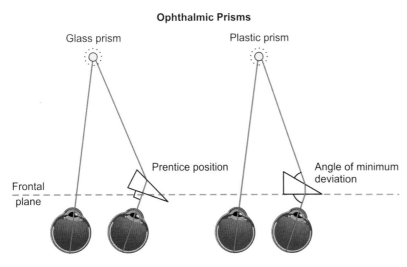

Fig. 7.11: Glass and plastic prisms are calibrated differently requiring them to be held in different positions. A glass prism must be held in the Prentice position, an orientation which causes light rays to strike one of the surfaces of the prism perpendicularly. An equally powered plastic prism, however, must be held parallel to the frontal plane such that the light bends equally at the two surfaces.

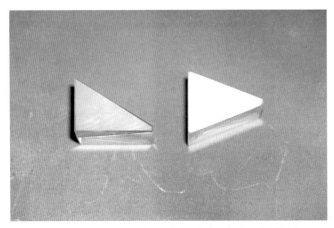

Fig. 7.12: 40 diopter glass (on left) and plastic (on right) prisms.

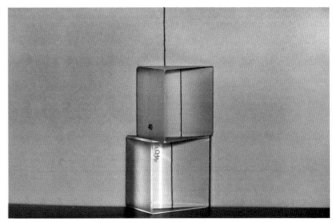

Fig. 7.13: For illustrative purposes the posterior surfaces of the 40 diopter glass and plastic prisms shown in Figure 7.12 have both been placed in the frontal plane. This is an incorrect position for the glass prism. Note that the deflection of light rays by these two prisms of equal power is quite different due to the incorrect positioning of the glass prism.

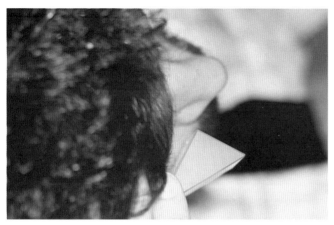

Fig. 7.14: The correct way to hold a glass prism for a patient with a left exotropia. The posterior surface of the glass prism must be held at 90° to the deviated eye's axis.

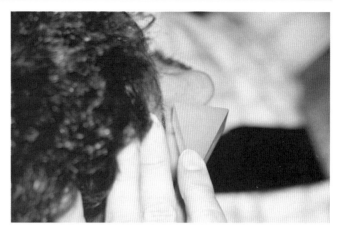

Fig. 7.15: The correct way to hold a plastic prism for a patient with a left exotropia. The posterior surface of a plastic prism must be held in the frontal plane.

ASSESSMENT OF OCULAR ALIGNMENT

Different types of tests are used to assess ocular alignment. These include corneal light reflex tests, cover tests, dissimilar image tests, dissimilar target tests and assessments of anatomic relationships.

Corneal Light Reflex Tests

Corneal light reflex tests use the image of incident light on the cornea to assess the status of ocular alignment. They are useful in patients who cannot cooperate for cover testing or who have poor fixation. Inherent to using corneal light reflex tests is an understanding of the normal reflection of a light source on the cornea and the angle kappa.

The Angle Kappa

The "angle kappa" (Figs 7.16A to C) is the angle formed between the visual axis and the pupillary axis. The "visual axis" is directed from the object of regard through the nodal point of the eye to the fovea. The "pupillary axis" connects the center of the pupil, perpendicular to the cornea, with the nodal point. Normally, the two do not correspond because the fovea is slightly temporally displaced. The corneal light reflex will normally be slightly nasal to the pupillary center. By definition, a nasally displaced corneal light reflex is termed a "positive angle kappa". A small positive angle kappa of up to 5° is physiologic.

A larger nasal displacement of the corneal light reflex mimics exotropia, and a temporal displacement, termed a "negative angle kappa", mimics esotropia. A large positive angle kappa, as seen in patients with cicatricial retinopathy

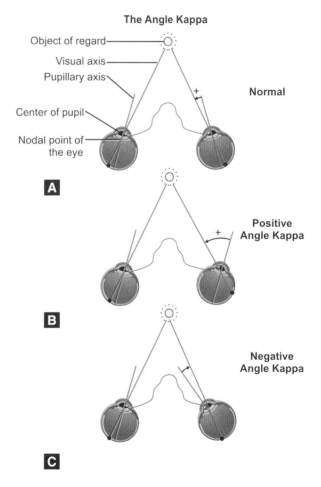

Figs 7.16A to C: (A) The angle formed between the visual and pupillary axes is the Angle Kappa. Normally the visual axis is slightly nasal to the pupillary axis, referred to as a small positive angle kappa; (B) In exotropia the angle kappa is a large positive angle; (C) In esotropia it is negative.

of prematurity with dragged maculas, may simulate an exodeviation (see section on pseudoexotropia in Chapter 9). Conversely, a large positive angle kappa may mask an esodeviation, and a negative angle kappa may mask an exodeviation.

Hirschberg's Light Reflex Test

Over 100 years ago, Hirschberg noted that when a patient fixated a light held 33 cm away, a 1-mm decentration of the corneal reflection of the light corresponded to 7° of deviation of the visual axes.[1] The corneal light reflex is normally slightly nasally displaced ("physiologic positive angle kappa"). A light reflex at the margin of a pupil 3.5–4.0 mm in size would be about 2 mm from the expected position and would correspond to 15° of deviation. A light reflex in the middle of the iris would equal 4 mm of decentration, or about 30° of deviation and at the limbus would equal 6 mm of decentration, or about 45° of deviation (Fig. 7.17).

Photographs can help document the decentered light reflex, as seen in progressively increasing esotropia (Figs 7.18A to D) and exotropia (Figs 7.19A to D), but Hirschberg's test is at best crude. Potential pitfalls include bilateral eccentric fixation and an abnormal angle kappa.

Krimsky's Test

Nearly fifty years ago, Krimsky described the use of prisms in front of the fixating eye to align the corneal light reflex in front of the deviating eye,[2] as shown for exotropic (Figs 7.20A and B) and hypotropic (Fig. 7.21) patients.

The optical basis of the test is shown in Figures 7.22A to C. A base-in prism placed in front of the fixating eye of a patient with exotropia causes the image in the retina of the fixating eye to be shifted nasally. The fixating eye will turn out to regain fixation. By Hering's law, the deviating eye makes a simultaneous and equal movement inward. Larger and larger prisms are introduced in front of the fixating eye until the corneal light reflex is centered on the deviating eye.

To correctly perform the test, the prism should be placed in front of the fixating eye, and the examiner should be seated directly in front of the deviating eye to avoid a parallax error in the estimation. The base of the prism

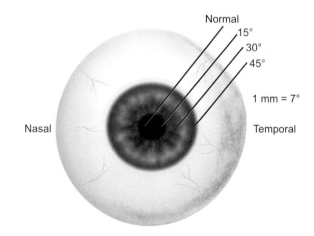

Left eye (pupil size = 3.5 mm)

Fig. 7.17: Hirschberg's light reflex test. A 1-mm decentration of the corneal reflection of the light correspondeds to approximately 7° of deviation of the visual axes.

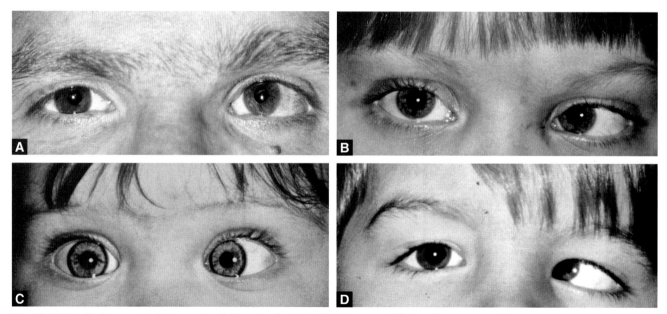

Figs 7.18A to D: Progressively increasing left esotropia. Note that the corneal light reflex progressively moves toward the temporal limbus of the eye.

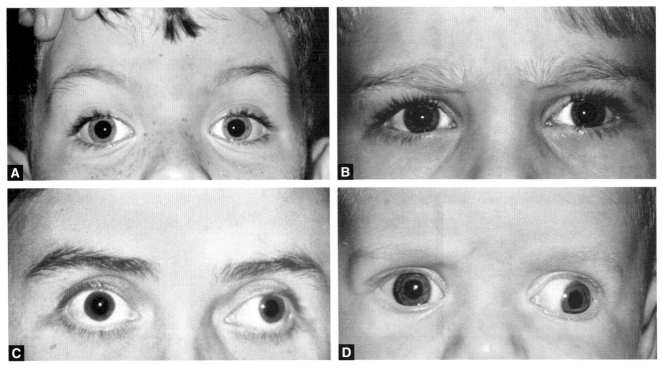

Figs 7.19A to D: Progressively increasing left exotropia. Note that the corneal light reflex progressively moves toward the nasal limbus of the eye.

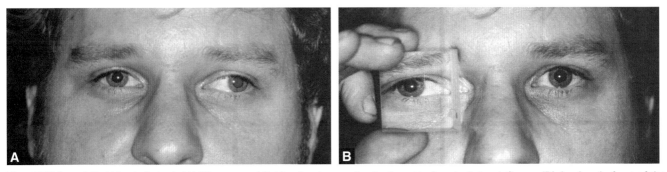

Figs 7.20A and B: Krimsky's test. (A) The corneal light reflex is nasally displaced in the deviating left eye; (B) A prism in front of the fixating right eye is used to center the corneal reflex.

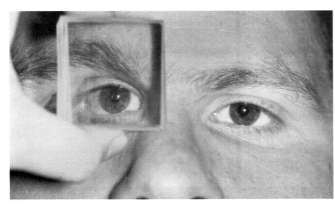

Fig. 7.21: Krimsky's test being performed on a patient with left hypotropia.

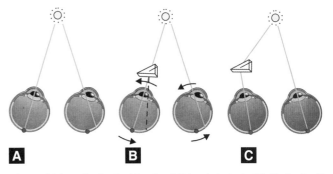

Figs 7.22A to C: Optical basis of Krimsky's test: (A) Patient with left exotropia; (B) A prism placed in front of the fixating left eye initially causes both eyes to rotate to the left; (C) The proper prism power will center the corneal light reflex on both corneas.

should always be opposite the direction of the deviation. For example, for esodeviations the base should be out; for exodeviations the base should be in. The deviation is recorded in prism diopters corresponding to the prism power needed to center the corneal light reflex in the deviating eye.

Estimation of the Corneal to Limbal Distance

In the strabismic patient with poor fixation and an opacified cornea, the corneal light reflex may be diffusely scattered and irregular. An alternative to the corneal light reflex test is an estimation of the canthal to limbal distance (Figs 7.23A and B). Larger and larger prisms are placed in front of the fixating eye until the distance between the canthus and the limbus in the deviated eye equals the same distance without prisms in the fixating eye.

Cover Tests

Cover tests provide an accurate and reproducible measure of ocular alignment. Prerequisites to cover testing include foveal fixation in each eye (Fig. 7.24), image perception from each eye, absence of restriction of eye movements, and patient cooperation. In addition, cover tests are based on a central alignment of the optics and retinas of the eyes. Any distortion of this such as occurs in patients with a dragged macula (Fig. 7.25) renders cover testing inaccurate in measuring any ocular misalignment that might be present. An error in the quantitation of the deviation will result.

All cover tests involve covering the apparently fixating eye. As shown in Figure 7.26, if an occluder is placed in front of the deviating eye, no ocular movement occurs.

The response to cover testing in both the occluded and the nonoccluded eye is observed. A previously fixating eye moves behind the occluder, a latent strabismus or phoria is

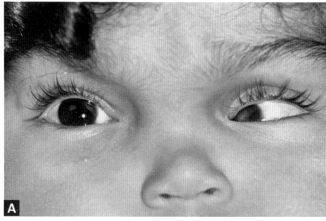 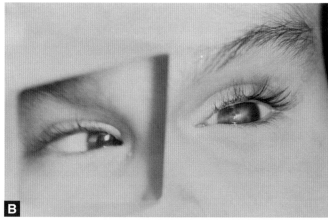

Figs 7.23A and B: Estimation of the Corneal to Limbal Distance: (A) Patient with a diffuse irregular scar on her left cornea; (B) With the use of a prism the distance from the canthus to the limbus in the deviating eye is equal to the same distance without prisms in fixating eye.

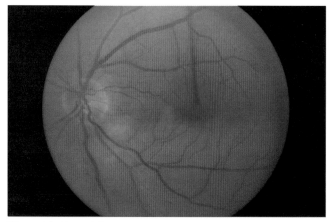 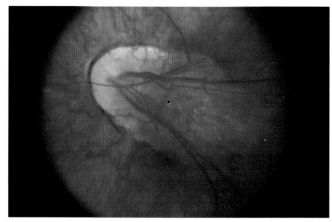

Fig. 7.24: Foveal fixation. The dark vertical band represents the fixation target which is centered on the fovea.

Fig. 7.25: Cover tests would be inaccurate in this patient with a dragged macula.

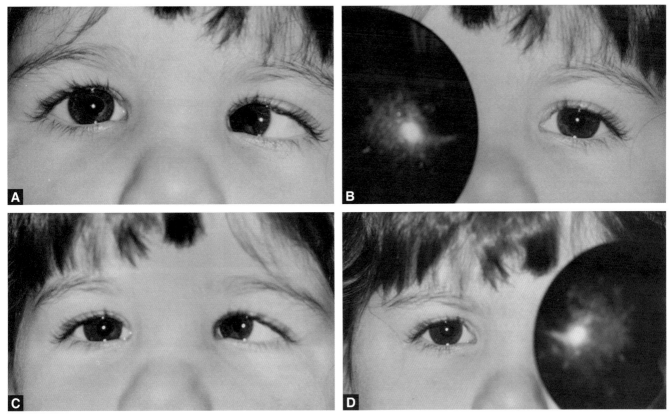

Figs 7.26A to D: Cover tests require that the fixating eye be covered: (A) Patient with left esotropia; (B) If an occluder is placed in front of the fixating right eye the left eye rotates outward to pick up fixation; (C) Same patient with left esotropia; (D) When the occluder is placed in front of the deviating left eye, no movement of right eye occurs.

present. If the nonoccluded eye rotates to pick up fixation, a manifest strabismus or tropia in the deviating eye is present.

There are three basic types of cover tests: the cover/uncover test, the alternate cover test and the simultaneous prism cover test.

The Cover/Uncover Test

The monocular cover/uncover test is useful in diagnosing and differentiating between phorias and tropias. If movement occurs behind the covered eye, a phoria is present. With phorias, the eyes are straight both before and after the cover/uncover test. Only when sensory fusion is interrupted does the occluded eye deviate (see Figs 7.1A and B). On first placing the occluder and interrupting fusion, the phoric eye drifts; a refixation movement in the opposite direction occurs when the cover is removed.

With tropias, however, one eye is already deviated prior to the test, and either the same eye (monocular strabismus) or the opposite eye (alternate strabismus) is deviated

at the end of the test. Figures 7.27 to 7.30 demonstrate the response to the cover/uncover test in various conditions.

If the patient has a nonalternating or monocular tropia, the deviation can be quantitated by introducing larger and larger prisms in front of the deviating eye until no refixation movement occurs on covering the initially fixating eye (Figs 7.31A to D).

The Alternate Cover Test

In the alternate cover (prism and cover) test, the cover is placed alternately in front of each eye, switching approximately every 2 seconds, to completely dissociate the eyes. Because simultaneous fixation by both eyes is not permitted, sensory fusion is eliminated, and any phoric component to the deviation is added to any tropic component. The total deviation, both latent and manifest, is obtained. Therefore, this test does not separate phorias from tropias, and it is not possible to specify how much of each is present.

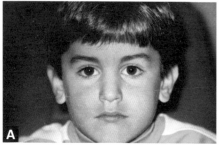
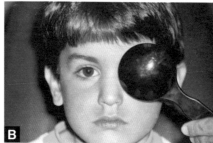
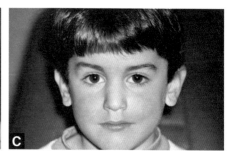

Figs 7.27A to C: The cover/uncover test in a child with orthophoria. No movement of either eye occurs upon covering an eye.

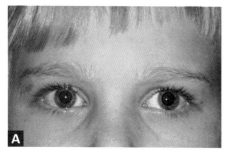
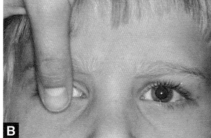
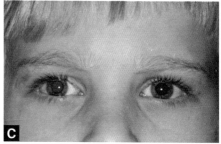

Figs 7.28A to C: The cover/uncover test in a patient with alternate exotropia. Upon covering the fixating right eye, the left eye picks up fixation and the right eye becomes exotropic.

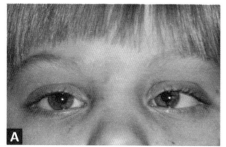
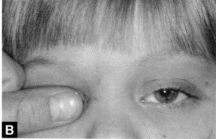
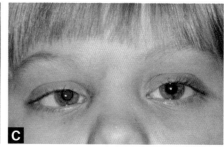

Figs 7.29A to C: The cover/uncover test in a patient with alternate esotropia. Upon covering the fixating right eye, the left eye picks up fixation and the right eye becomes esotropic.

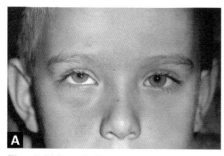
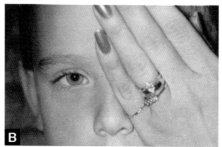
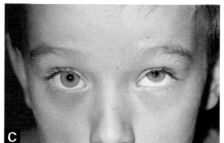

Figs 7.30A to C: The cover/uncover test in a patient with alternate hypertropia. Upon covering the fixating left eye, the right eye picks up fixation and the left eye becomes hypertropic.

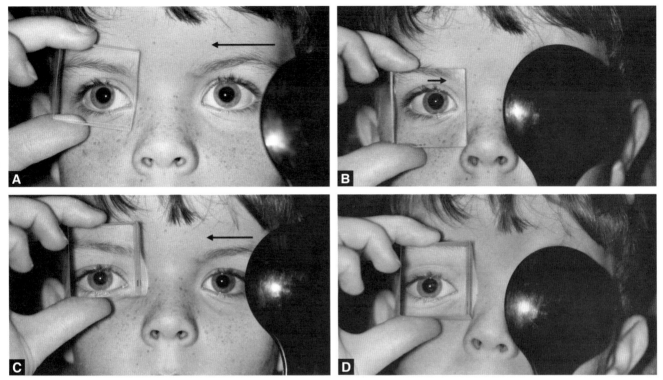

Figs 7.31A to D: Quantitation of a tropia using the cover/uncover test and larger and larger prisms in a patient with a monocular right exotropia. (A) With a small prism held in front of the deviating right eye a cover is introduced in front of the fixating left eye; (B) Because the prism in front of the right eye was not large enough the right eye moves inward to pick up fixation when the left eye is occluded; (C) A larger prism is placed in front of the right eye and the occluder is reintroduced in front of the fixating left eye; (D) With the larger prism there is no movement of the right eye when the left eye is occluded. The deviation has been quantitated.

Once the eyes are completely dissociated and the total deviation is manifest, larger and larger prisms are placed in front of one eye until no movement occurs as the cover is alternated from one eye to the other. The prism power necessary to completely eliminate any refixation movement by the nonoccluded eye is the amount of total deviation (Figs 7.32A to F). Prisms always shift the image in the direction of the base of the prism. Base-out prisms are used for esotropia, base-in prisms for exotropia, base-down prisms for hypertropia, and base-up prisms for hypotropia. The test is carried out at both near and distant fixation.

The Simultaneous Prism and Cover Test

The simultaneous prism and cover test allows the examiner to quantitate the tropic component of a deviation that has a superimposed phoric component. This test does not dissociate the eyes; it allows sensory fusion to keep in abeyance the phoric component.

The test is performed by simultaneously introducing a prism in front of the deviating eye and an occluder in front of the fixating eye. If movement occurs in the eye behind the prism, the end point has not been reached. Both cover and prism are removed, and larger prisms are chosen until no shift occurs in the deviated eye, as shown in Figures 7.33A to C. The tropic component of the deviation is thus quantitated because sensory fusion is allowed at all times just prior to introducing the prism and cover.

This test is especially useful in the "monofixation syndrome", in which patients may reduce the total deviation (as measured by the alternate cover and cover/uncover tests) by using peripheral sensory fusion to partially control a coexisting phoria. As shown in Figures 7.33D to F, using the same size prism that neutralized the deviation with the simultaneous prism cover test, a refixation movement occurs with the cover/uncover test. A larger prism (Figs 7.33G to I) is needed to neutralize the deviation, using the cover/uncover test.

Dissimilar Image Tests

Dissimilar image tests quantitate ocular deviations by first creating dissimilar images for the two eyes that the patient

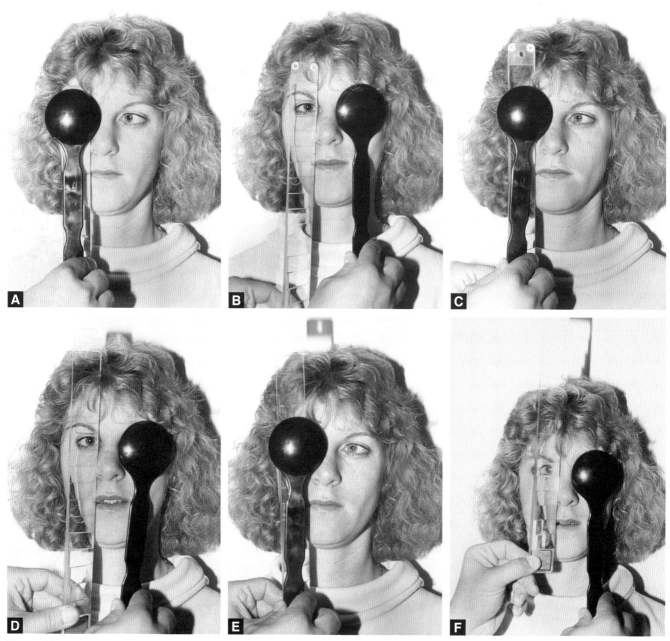

Figs 7.32A to F: The alternate cover (prism and cover) test: Larger and larger prisms are placed in front of one eye until no movement in either eye occurs as the occluder is alternated between the two eyes. The prism power needed to completely eliminate refixation equals the amount of total deviation.

can appreciate and then superimposing the images by the use of prisms. The two major instruments that are used to create dissimilar images are the red glass filter and the Maddox rod. The red glass test is described under sensory adaptations to strabismus (see Figs 6.4 and 6.5). The Maddox rod provides two additional tests.

The Optical Basis of Maddox Rod Testing

A Maddox rod is a series of high-powered plus-cylinder lenses aligned so that their axes are parallel. When light rays from a point source strike a plus-cylinder lens the rays are refracted to form a line image parallel to the axis of the cylinder (Fig. 7.34, *top).* This real image lies behind

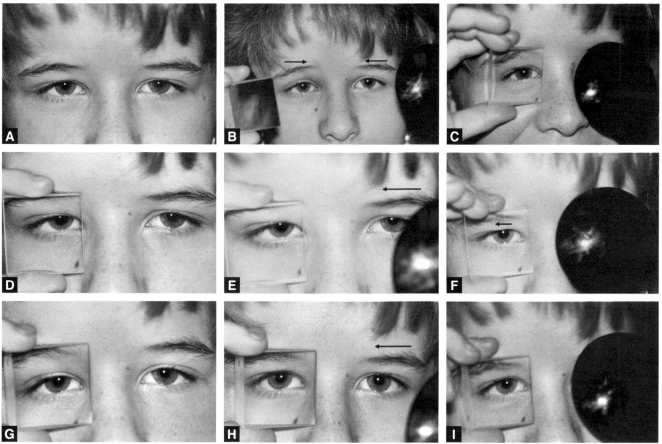

Figs 7.33A to I: The simultaneous prism and cover test in a patient with the Monofixation Syndrome: (A to C) The simultaneous prism and cover test is performed by simultaneously introducing a prism in front of the deviating eye and an occluder in front of the fixating eye. In this patient, this elicited 20 diopters of esotropia. (D to F) This patient's total deviation, however, is larger than 20 diopters. When a cover/uncover test is performed using the same 20 diopter prism that neutralized the deviation in the simultaneous prism and cover test (above) additional esotropia is elicited. (G to I) A larger prism (in this case 30 diopters) is needed to neutralize the deviation using the cover/uncover test. This patient with Monofixation Syndrome uses peripheral sensory fusion to reduce the total deviation.

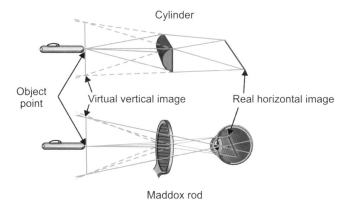

Fig. 7.34: The Maddox rod: (Top) Light rays from a point source are refracted to form a real line image parallel to the axis of the cylinder in front of the rod and a perpendicular virtual line image at the light source. (Bottom) Optics of the Maddox rod test and the eye.

the cylinder. Because the light rays were converged by the cylinder, one can artificially extend the rays backward (dotted lines) to construct a virtual but perceivable image of the point source. The virtual image is also a line, but it is oriented at 90° to the real image. It passes directly through the point source of light, and therefore is located in front of the cylinder.

When a horizontally oriented cylinder is placed in front of an eye, a real horizontal image is formed just behind the lens of the eye (Fig. 7.34, *bottom*). This real image is too close to the retina to be focused and will not be appreciated. The vertical virtual image, however, lies in front of the eye at the object point. It can be focused and imaged on the retina. A plus cylinder creates two images, but only the virtual line image oriented at 90° to the axis of the cylinder is seen. A Maddox rod is simply a series of aligned plus cylinders stacked together to make the virtual vertical line image appear larger. For even greater contrast a red Maddox rod can be used.

The Single Maddox Rod Test

To perform this test, a Maddox rod is either held by the patient or placed in a trial frame or phoroptor in front of one eye. On viewing a bright light, a line will be imaged on the patient's retina oriented at 90° to the axis of the cylinders that compose the Maddox rod. For the patient shown in Figures 7.35A and B the ridges of the Maddox rod (axes of the cylinders) are oriented vertically. A horizontal line will be imaged on his right retina.

The response sought in the single Maddox rod test is where the line imaged by the eye behind the Maddox rod is located in relation to the light source imaged by the other eye (Fig. 7.36A). In orthophoria the patient reports that the line intersects the point light source regardless of how the Maddox rod is oriented. To test for horizontal deviations, the Maddox rod needs to be oriented with its ridges horizontally to form a vertical image on the retina. In esotropia, the line is imaged on the nasal retina and is perceived to be located temporally or on the same side as the Maddox rod (uncrossed diplopia). The opposite is true for exotropia. To test for vertical deviations, the Maddox rod needs to be oriented with its ridges vertical, to form a horizontal line image on the retina. In hypotropia, the line is imaged on the inferior retina and is perceived to be above the light source. The opposite occurs with hypertropia.

To quantitate the deviation, prisms are introduced in front of the Maddox rod (Fig. 7.36B). The Maddox rod test is a dissociative test because it forms dissimilar images that cannot be fused. Sensory fusion cannot reduce the disparity of the images, and the total deviation, both phoric and tropic, will be elicited. The total deviation equals the prism power used to center the line.

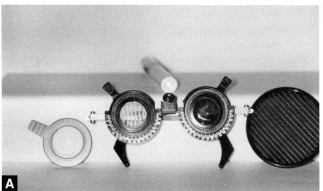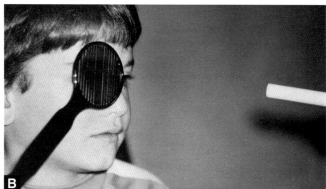

Figs 7.35A and B: Maddox rod test: (A) Flashlight and different Maddox rods that can be used including red and white rods and rods that fit inside trial frames or an occluder; (B) Test being performed. In this patient, the ridges of the Maddox rod (axes of the cylinders) are oriented vertically, therefore a virtual horizontal line will be perceived by the patient.

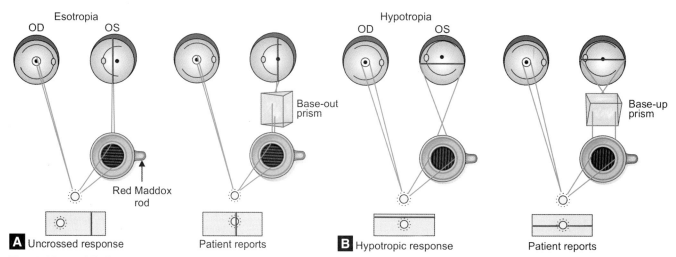

Figs 7.36A and B: Results reported on Maddox rod testing. (A) A patient with a left esotropia will report that the line image is to the left of the light (uncrossed). A base-out prism of the proper power aligns the line with the light; (B) A patient with left hypotropia will report that the line image is above the light. A base-up prism of the proper power aligns the line with the light.

To review, horizontal deviations are measured with the ridges of the Maddox rod oriented horizontally, and vertical deviations are measured with the ridges oriented vertically. The Maddox rod creates an image on the retina oriented 90° to its axis, a vertical line for horizontal deviations and a horizontal line for vertical deviations. Prisms are used to shift the vertical line image horizontally for horizontal deviations, and vertically for vertical deviations. The base of the prism is placed in the direction in which one wants to move the image, which also corresponds to the direction away from the point source from which the line is seen.

This test should not be used to quantitate horizontal deviations at near fixation because accommodative convergence cannot be controlled with this test.

The Double Maddox Rod Test

When two Maddox rods of different colors (usually red and white) are used in conjunction, each in front of one eye, cyclodeviations can be measured.

The Maddox rods can be placed in either a trial frame or a phoroptor, both directed so that their axes are exactly vertical in order to create a horizontal line image for each eye from a point light source. A small base-down prism in front of one eye separates the images and helps prevent sensory cyclofusion, facilitating the recognition of two separate lines. If the patient reports that the two lines are not parallel, a cyclodeviation exists. The patient is then asked to rotate the axis of one or both of the Maddox rods to make the lines horizontal and parallel to each other. The cyclodeviation is quantitated in degrees from a scale on the trial frames or phoroptor. The direction of the deviation (incyclotropia or excyclotropia) is determined by noting the direction in which the top of the Maddox rod (the 12:00 meridian) is rotated. An inward rotation corresponds with an incyclotropia, and an outward rotation corresponds with an excyclotropia. The patient shown in Figures 7.37A to C has a left superior oblique palsy. The red line image is seen as intorted. In order to align the two lines the red Maddox rod has to be rotated outward, indicating that the patient has an excyclotropia (Figs 7.38A and B).

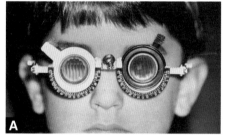
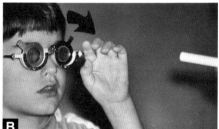
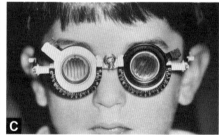

Figs 7.37A to C: The Double Maddox rod test. (A) White and red Maddox rods are respectively placed in front of the right and left eyes using a trial frame; (B) While viewing a penlight the child with a cyclodeviation is asked to rotate one or both of the lenses so that the lines are both horizontal; (C) The resultant cyclodeviation is then able to be quantitated in degrees.

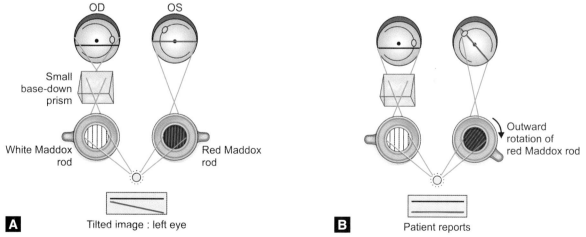

Figs 7.38A and B: The Double Maddox rod test in a patient with a left superior oblique (LSO) palsy. (A) Secondary to the LSO palsy the patient's left eye is excyclotropic. He reports seeing the red line intorted; (B) The red Maddox rod is outwardly rotated (excyclotorted) until the patient reports that the red and white lines are parallel. Note that a small prism has been placed in front of the fixating right eye so that the images of the red and white light are not superimposed and can better be appreciated by the patient as parallel lines.

Topographic Relationship between the Optic Nerve and the Fovea

Sensory cyclofusion of up to 10–15° can be well developed in congenital cyclodeviations, rendering subjective cyclotorsion testing (the double Maddox rod test) inaccurate at times. Motor cyclofusion, however, is rarely well developed, and rotation of the fundus about the antero-posterior axis can still be visualized by ophthalmoscopy.

Anatomically, the fovea is located about one third of a disk diameter below the center of the optic nerve (Fig. 7.39). In cyclodeviations, the optic nerve is rotated in relation to the fovea. With incyclodeviations the optic nerve is lower than the fovea (Fig. 7.40), and with excyclodeviations the optic nerve is higher (Fig. 7.41).

The indirect ophthalmoscope inverts and reverses the image of the retina seen by the observer. As opposed to the view with the direct ophthalmoscope and fundus camera, when viewing the fundus through an indirect ophthalmoscope if the optic nerve is higher than the fovea, intorsion of the fundus exists (Fig. 7.42). If the optic nerve is lower than the fovea when viewed through the indirect ophthalmoscope, extorsion of the retina exists (Fig. 7.43).

Dissimilar Target Tests

Dissimilar image tests (see previous section) create different images for the two eyes, which the examiner then superimposes for the patient using prisms. "Dissimilar target tests" provide different targets for the two eyes that the patient is asked to superimpose. The former tests create an awareness of misaligned images that are then aligned using prisms. The latter tests dissociate the eyes and record the perceived spatial location of the object of regard for each eye separately. Dissimilar target tests record where the image from the fovea of each eye is projected and therefore are useful primarily for patients with normal retinal correspondence. These tests first locate a target with one eye and then ask where a dissimilar target for the other eye must lie in space if the two targets are to be superimposed. Dissimilar target tests are useful in incomitant paralytic strabismus to determine the position of gaze in which the maximum deviation occurs and to demonstrate the inequity of primary and secondary deviations.

The major dissimilar target tests used are the major amblyoscope and Lees', Hess', and Lancaster's screen tests. The major amblyoscope is discussed under sensory adaptations to strabismus (see Chapter 6). In all the screen tests, the examiner projects or indicates a spot on a ruled screen that only one eye of the patient can see. The patient

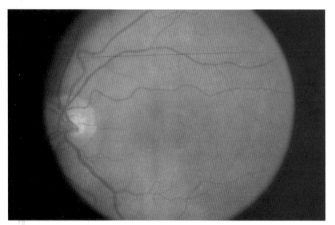

Fig. 7.39: Normal appearance of the left fundus through the direct ophthalmoscope. The fovea is seen about one third of a disk diameter below the center of the optic nerve.

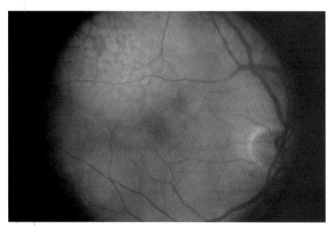

Fig. 7.40: Appearance of the right fundus through the direct ophthalmoscope when the eye is incyclodeviated. The optic nerve is lower than the fovea.

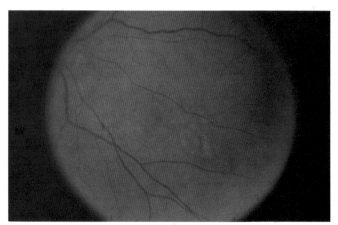

Fig. 7.41: Appearance of the left fundus through the direct ophthalmoscope when the eye is excyclodeviated. The optic nerve is higher than the fovea.

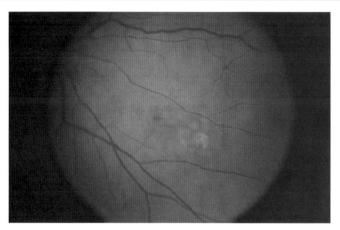

Fig. 7.42: Appearance of the right fundus through the indirect ophthalmoscope when the eye is incyclodeviated. The optic nerve is higher than the fovea.

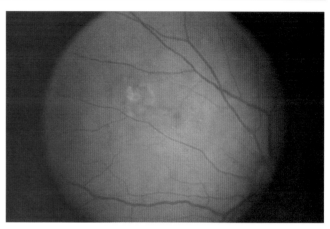

Fig. 7.43: Appearance of the left fundus through the indirect ophthalmoscope when the eye is excyclodeviated. The optic nerve is lower than the fovea.

is then asked to project or indicate where a target seen by the other eye would lie if it were to superimpose the target of the first eye. By repeating this for the cardinal positions of gaze, the gaze position of maximal deviation can be identified. The results are recorded on miniaturized charts that replicate the screen used. For Lees' and Hess' screen tests, the points found are connected by straight lines, permitting the examiner to determine which muscles act abnormally. Primary deviations are recorded when the dominant eye fixates the first target. Secondary deviations are recorded by allowing the eye with the paretic muscle to fixate the first target.

Figure 7.44 shows "Lees' screen test" being performed. This test uses two screens oriented at 90° to each other. The patient sits directly in front of one screen, which is viewed by his left eye. A mirror angled at 45° projects the second screen to his right eye. The examiner provides targets to one eye using the first screen, and the patient uses the other screen to indicate where a superimposed target for the other eye lies. Figure 7.45 shows the chart used to record the results. The smaller field, which results when the dominant eye is fixating, represents the primary deviation and indicates where a superimposed target for the eye with the palsied muscle(s) lies, therefore identifying the eye with the paretic muscle. This field is then examined to ascertain in which cardinal position of gaze the displacement away from the normal position is greatest. The muscle acting in this position of gaze is the palsied one. In this example, the left inferior rectus muscle is paretic.

"Hess' screen test" is based on the same principles as those of Lees' screen test but uses only one black screen

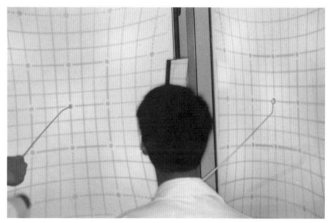

Fig. 7.44: Lee's (dissimilar target) test being performed. The examiner presents targets to one eye and the patient indicates where a superimposed target for the other eye lies.

on which are fixed red dots corresponding to the cardinal positions of gaze and over which a movable Y-shaped configuration of green cords slides. The patient wears red and green goggles and is asked to superimpose the red dots seen with one eye with the green cords seen only with the other eye. The results are recorded in exactly the same manner as with Lees' screen test.

"Lancaster's screen test" also uses red and green glasses, but in this test the targets for the two eyes are projected onto the screen, which again can be directed into the cardinal positions of gaze. A useful feature of this test is that a line target can be projected and the amount of cyclotorsion that exists in each of the cardinal positions of gaze can be compared.

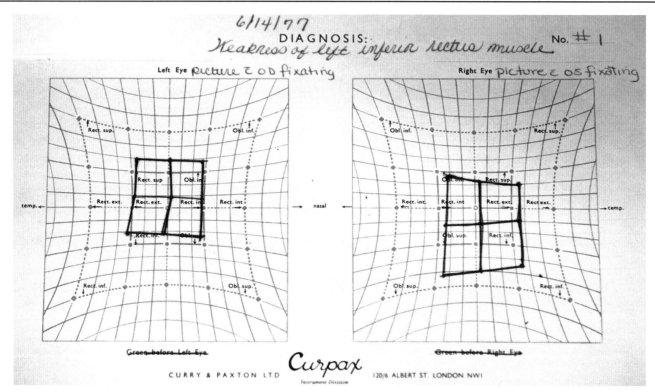

Fig. 7.45: Chart used to record the results of a Lee's screen test. In this patient, a palsy of the left inferior rectus muscle was identified because a smaller field was mapped with the nonparetic right eye fixating (left side of the chart) and the deviation was greatest in the direction of action of the inferior rectus.

SPECIAL TESTS AND TECHNIQUES IN THE ASSESSMENT OF OCULAR ALIGNMENT

Diplopia Visual Fields

Using either a Goldmann's perimeter or a tangent screen, a small white test object is followed by both eyes together throughout the visual field (Figs 7.46A and B). The entire visual field is plotted, noting areas of single vision and double vision. This test is useful diagnostically and can be repeated at later dates to substantiate the results of therapy or time.

Forced Duction Testing

In a forced duction test, the anesthetized eye is mechanically moved into various positions of gaze to detect any resistance to passive movement. Resistance to passive movement is considered a "positive" result.

The test is best performed by grasping conjunctiva and episclera near the limbus with two forceps held 180° apart (Figs 7.47A to D). The eye is moved into positions suspected of being restricted as a result of mechanical

factors. Care must be exercised not to press the globe into the orbit, as this may give false-negative results in the face of true restriction. When the test is done using topical anesthesia, the patient is asked to look in the direction the eye is being moved to eliminate any resistance caused by extraocular muscle contraction in the opposite direction. This test is most useful in differentiating restrictive from paretic disorders.

Active Force Generation Testing

The active force generation test is helpful in determining the residual function of paretic muscles. With the eye stabilized with a forceps (Fig. 7.48), the patient is asked to move her eye in the opposite direction. For a patient with a right superior rectus palsy the forceps is placed at the inferior limbus, and the patient is asked to look up. If the examiner detects a tug on the forceps, some residual function of the right superior rectus exists. It is important to place the forceps at 180° to the direction of the intended movement because if the forceps is placed in the path of intended movement, slippage of the forceps could result in a corneal abrasion.

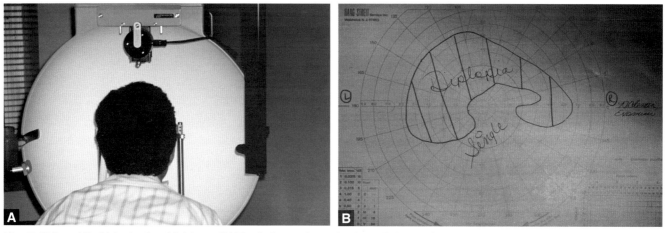

Figs 7.46A and B: Diplopia visual field test. (A) Test being performed using a Goldmann's perimeter; (B) Results of test indicating where in the visual field the patient's vision is single versus double.

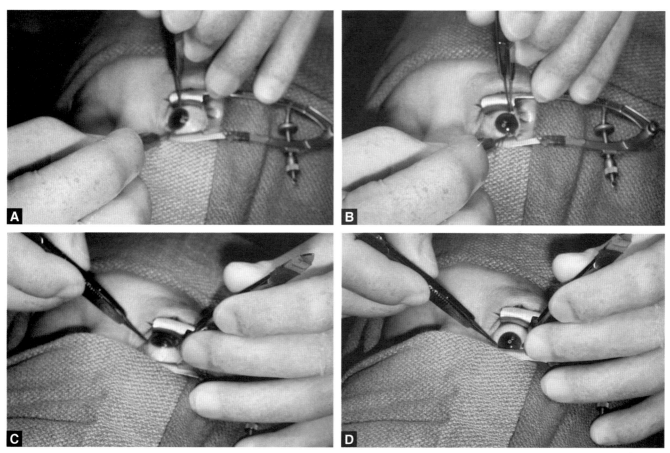

Figs 7.47A to D: Forced duction testing. The eye is moved in the cardinal positions of gaze (A) Adduction; (B) Abduction; (C) Elevation; (D) Depression.

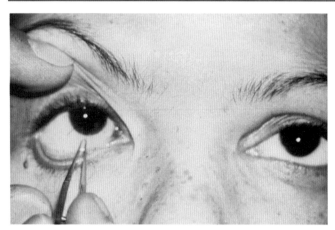

Fig. 7.48: Active Force Generation Testing. With the eye stabilized with a forceps the patient is asked to move her eye in the opposite direction.
Courtesy: Joseph H Calhoun MD.

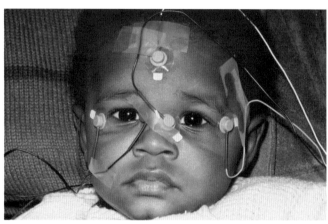

Fig. 7.49: Child with electro-oculographic apparatus positioned to test saccadic velocities.

Saccadic Velocity Testing

Saccadic velocity testing is another useful test to differentiate paretic from restrictive disorders. It is especially useful in infants in whom forced duction testing would require general anesthesia.

Using electro-oculographic apparatus (Fig. 7.49), electric recordings of the speed of voluntary eye movements can be registered by directing the patient's gaze to desired positions. The velocity of the saccade, starting from the opposite position of gaze and ending at the desired position of gaze, remains normal in restrictive disorders despite the limited excursion of the eye.

The Three-Step Test to Diagnose Cyclovertical Muscle Palsies

Patients with an acute palsy of one of the eight cyclovertical muscles will have a manifest hypertropia. In 1958, Parks described a method, based on Hofmann and Bielschowsky's head tilt test of 1900, that uses three steps to identify which of the eight cyclovertical muscles is paretic in patients with an isolated, acute cyclovertical muscle palsy.[3] This test is useful only when all of the three conditions he enumerated are present. The muscle involved must be paretic, it must be the only paretic muscle, and it must be one of the muscles that have cyclovertical action. This test is not useful when more than one muscle is palsied or when a restrictive disorder is present. The three-step test cannot be used to isolate paretic horizontally acting muscles.

Each step in the three-step test progressively halves the possible choices, so that at the end of the third step, only one muscle remains, which must be the paretic muscle. The first step reduces the possible choices from eight to four muscles simply by looking at which eye is higher.

The second step reduces the possible choices to two by determining whether the deviation is worse in right gaze or in left gaze. The second step is based on the fact that different muscles act in right and left gaze. The third step identifies the one paretic muscle. This step utilizes the utricular reflex that occurs on tilting the head (Fig. 7.50). This otolith response serves to keep the eyes vertically and cyclotorsionally aligned by rotating or torting the eyes about the anteroposterior axis in a direction opposite the head rotation. If the head is tilted to the right, the utricular reflex stimulates the right superior oblique and right superior rectus muscles to incycloduct the right eye. The corresponding movement of the left eye is excycloduction brought about by contracture of the left inferior oblique and left inferior rectus muscles. The opposite occurs with a left head tilt. In this manner, the eyes remain vertically and cyclotorsionally aligned when the head is tilted.

To facilitate understanding of the test, separate illustrations are used for patients with right and left hypertropias (Figs 7.51 and 7.52). Below each set of eyes is a listing of the four cyclovertical muscles of each eye in an order that corresponds to the position of gaze for which each muscle acts as the prime mover of the eye. For instance, the elevators of the eye are the superior rectus and inferior oblique muscles. They are listed above the inferior rectus and superior oblique, which are depressors of the eye. The vertical rectus muscles are the prime movers of the eye in the abducted position, and the oblique muscles act when the eye is adducted. The rectus muscles are therefore listed on the outside, and the oblique muscles are listed on the inside. Use of this notation to record the responses on the three-step test helps to isolate the one paretic muscle.

Head Tilt

Right head tilt | Left head tilt

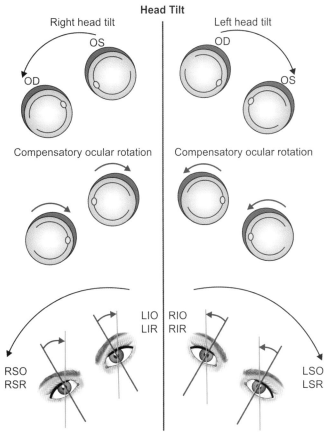

Compensatory ocular rotation | Compensatory ocular rotation

LIO | RIO
LIR | RIR

RSO
RSR

LSO
LSR

Fig. 7.50: Physiologic basis of the Three-Step Test. Upon tilting the head a utricular reflex occurs which serves to keep the eyes vertically and cyclotorsionally aligned. If the head is tilted to the right, the right superior oblique (RSO) and right superior rectus (RSR) muscles incycloduct the right eye and the left inferior oblique (LIO) and left inferior rectus (LIR) muscles excycloduct the left eye. With left head tilt the right inferior oblique (RIO) and right inferior rectus (RIR) muscles excycloduct the right eye and the left superior oblique (LSO) and left superior rectus (LSR) muscles incycloduct the left eye.

The Three-Step Test for Right Hypertropia (Fig. 7.51)

Step I: The first step involves determining which eye is higher. In this instance, the right eye is higher than the left eye. This means that the paretic muscle must be one that either depresses the right eye or elevates the left eye. Of the eight cyclovertical muscles, the muscles that depress the right eye are the right inferior rectus (RIR) and the right superior oblique (RSO). The muscles that elevate the left eye are the left inferior oblique (LIO) and the left superior rectus (LSR). One of these four muscles must be paretic if the right eye is higher than the left eye. These muscles are circled in Figure 7.51. This step reduces the possible paretic muscles from eight to four.

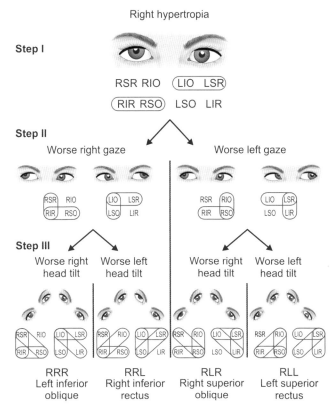

Fig. 7.51: The three-step test for right hypertropia. In each step the potential palsied muscle is circled. At the end of Step III only one muscle has been circled three times, identifying it as the palsied muscle.

Step II: The second step determines whether the vertical deviation is greater in right or left gaze. If the deviation is worse in right gaze (Fig. 7.51, *left),* the paretic muscle must be one of the four that is used in right gaze. In the right eye, these are the right superior rectus (RSR) and RIR. For the left eye, the muscles that act in right gaze are the LIO and left superior oblique (LSO). These muscles are circled in Figure 7.51. The same can be done if the deviation is worse in left gaze (Fig. 7.51, *right).* At the end of the second step, for any possible paresis, only two muscles have been circled twice, reducing the possible choices for the paretic muscle from four to two.

Step III: The third step of the three-step test determines whether the vertical deviation is worse on right or left head tilt. As shown in Figure 7.50, on right head tilt the RSR and right superior oblique (RSO) contract to incycloduct the right eye, and the LIO and left inferior rectus (LIR) contract to excycloduct the left eye. On left head tilt the stimulated muscles are the RIR and RIO to excycloduct the right eye, and the LSR and LSO to incycloduct the left eye. Depending on whether the vertical misalignment is worse on right or left head tilt, the muscles that are used respectively are circled in Figure 7.51. For every possibility only one muscle is circled three times. This muscle is the isolated paretic muscle. Below each diagram are the abbreviated results. For example, a left inferior oblique palsy is present when the "right" hypertropia is worse on "right" gaze and "right" head tilt *(RRR)*.

The Three-Step Test for Left Hypertropia (Fig. 7.52)

Step I: If the left eye is higher than the right eye, the possible paretic muscles (circled) are the elevators of the right eye, the RSR or the RIO, or the depressors of the left eye, the LSO or the LIR.

Step II: If the deviation is worse in right gaze, the muscles that act in this gaze, the RSR, RIR, LIO and LSO, are circled. The RIO, RSO, LSR and LIR are circled if the deviation is worse in left gaze. At the end of this step, only two possible choices for the paretic muscle remain for a patient with a left hypertropia worse in right gaze. They are the only muscles circled twice in Figure 7.52, the RSR or LSO. For the patient with a left hypertropia worse in left gaze, either the RIO or the LIR must be palsied.

Step III: The final step identifies the paretic muscle in patients with a left hypertropia. If the deviation is worse on right gaze and right head tilt, the RSR is identified. If the deviation is worse on right gaze and left head tilt, the LSO is paretic (Also see Figs 11.8 and 11.9). For the patient with a left hypertropia worse on left gaze and right head tilt the LIR is identified. If the hypertropia is worse on left gaze and left head tilt, the RIO must be paretic.

▪ ABNORMAL HEAD POSITIONS

Abnormal head positions can occur with skeletal or muscular abnormalities of the head and neck; with paresis or restriction of an ocular muscle; and in association with congenital nystagmus, strabismus syndromes, and ptosis.

Nonocular Causes of Abnormal Head Positions

Nonocular causes of abnormal head positions ("torticollis") include congenital bony malformations of the cervical vertebrae or abnormalities of the sternocleidomastoid or trapezius muscles. The patient in Figure 7.53 had multiple muscular and bony abnormalities, including a tight left trapezius muscle (Fig. 7.54) causing a constant left head tilt.

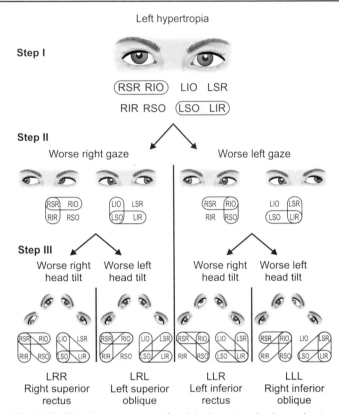

Fig. 7.52: The three-step test for right hypertropia. In each step the potential palsied muscle is circled. At the end of Step III only one muscle has been circled three times, identifying it as the palsied muscle.

To differentiate a head tilt caused by skeletal or muscular abnormalities from that caused by an ocular misalignment, a "patch test" can be performed. The eye with the suspected paretic muscle is occluded (Figs 7.55A and B). If the head tilt disappears on occluding this eye, as in this patient with a superior oblique palsy, the ocular cause of the head tilt is confirmed.

Congenital Nystagmus

Patients with congenital nystagmus often demonstrate a dampening of the amplitude of their nystagmus in a specific direction of gaze called the "null point" or "neutral zone" of the nystagmus. Their visual acuity may be better with their eyes in the null position. A patient with nystagmus whose null point is an eccentric position of gaze will turn his or her head to position the eyes in this eccentric position of gaze (Fig. 7.56A) to obtain the best visual acuity. Sometimes, a compromise is made between the best visual acuity and the noticeable cosmetic appearance of a large face turn, as in this patient who foregoes his best vision for a less noticeable, smaller face turn (Fig. 7.56B).

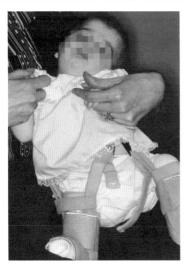

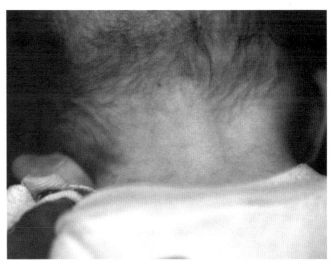

Fig. 7.53: Torticollis secondary to multiple muscular and bony abnormalities, including a tight left trapezius muscle.

Fig. 7.54: Tight left trapezius muscle in the child in Figure 7.53 causing a constant left head tilt.

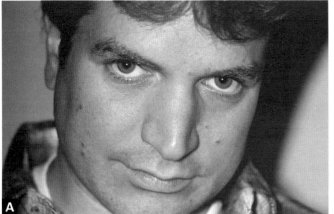

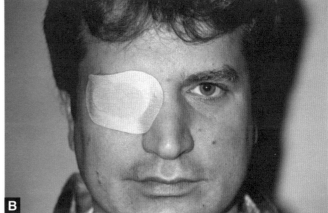

Figs 7.55A and B: Patch test used to differentiate a head tilt secondary to a skeletal or muscular abnormality from that due to an ocular misalignment. In this patient, the head tilt (A) disappears on occluding his right eye confirming the diagnosis of a right superior oblique palsy.

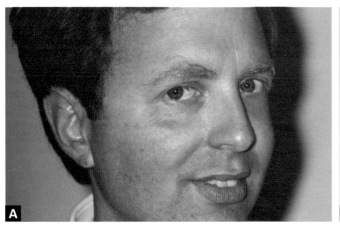

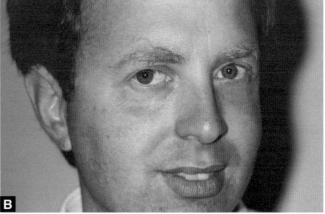

Figs 7.56A and B: Head turn in a patient with nystagmus. (A) The null point for this patient is in far right gaze; (B) The same patient in his typical resting position. He has compromised his best vision for a less noticeable, smaller head turn.

■ OCULAR MUSCLE PARESES AND RESTRICTIONS

Patients with acute ocular motor paresis or restriction often tilt their heads, turn their faces, or elevate or depress their chins to prevent horizontal, vertical, or cyclotorsional diplopia. The abnormal head position places the eyes in a position in which the paretic or restricted muscle does not need to function. Rarely, patients who cannot achieve single vision in any position of gaze will turn their heads in such a way as to maximize the separation of the two images, making the diplopia more tolerable.

The use of head position to diagnose ocular muscle paresis or restrictions is fraught with possible errors and limitations. Variable hypertrophy or secondary contracture of the direct antagonist of the paretic muscle or overaction of its yoke muscle may lead to a head position different from the position expected. Secondary structural changes in the cervical spine and muscles of the neck may result in the persistence of torticollis after surgical correction of the ocular misalignment, or the torticollis may persist out of

habit. Furthermore, the absence of torticollis does not rule out a cyclovertical muscle abnormality. With respect for the limitations of this evaluation the following observations can be made.

Face Turns

With a horizontal rectus muscle paresis or restriction or with Duane's syndrome the face is turned in such a way as to place the eyes out of the field of action of the abnormal muscle. If the right medial rectus muscle is palsied or restricted, the face is turned to the opposite or left side so that the right eye is in the abducted position, as seen in Figures 7.57A to D. This patient has myositis of the right medial rectus muscle. He is orthophoric in right gaze (Fig. 7.57A) but progressively more exotropic in left gaze (Figs 7.57 B and C). To avoid diplopia, he developed a left face turn (Fig. 7.57 D). The patient with paresis or restriction of the lateral rectus muscle turns his or her head to the ipsilateral side to place the eye with the paretic lateral rectus muscle in the adducted position (Also see Fig. 8.19).

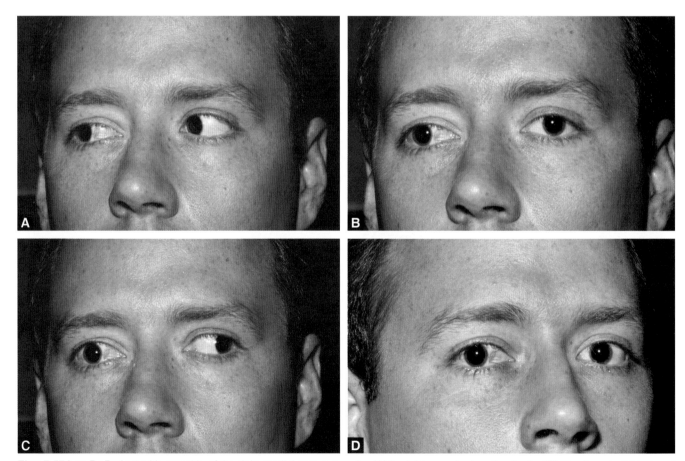

Figs 7.57A to D: Patient with myositis of the right medial rectus muscle. (A) In right gaze he is orthophoric; (B) Fixating straight ahead he has a small right exotropia; (C) In left gaze, he has a large right exotropia; (D) To avoid diplopia, he developed a left face turn.

Head Tilts with Face Turns

The patient with a cyclovertical muscle palsy may tilt his or her head to eliminate cyclovertical and vertical diplopia. This head tilt is usually accompanied by a face turn and a chin elevation or depression. Torticollis is more common and more characteristic with oblique muscle palsies. With palsies of the oblique muscles, the head often points toward the defect allowing the eyes to move in the opposite direction. With vertical rectus muscle palsies the head can be tilted to either the involved or the opposite side, depending on whether the yoke of the underacting muscle is overacting or if there is contraction of the direct antagonist of the paretic muscle. The face turn and chin position are more consistent and can be thought of as having the effect of placing the eye out of the position of action of the paretic muscle.

The classic head position for a patient with a right superior oblique muscle palsy is a head tilt and face turn to the opposite side and depression of the chin (Fig. 7.58). Tilting the head to the left calls on the right eye to excycloduct (see Fig. 7.50), which requires the RIO and RIR, but not the RSO, to contract. The left face turn and chin depression also place the eye out of the field of action for this muscle.

The usual position for a right inferior oblique muscle palsy is an ipsilateral head tilt, a contralateral face turn and chin elevation (Fig. 7.59). On right head tilt the right eye is called on to incycloduct, which requires the actions of the RSR and RSO, but not the RIO. The left face turn and chin elevation also place the eye out of the position of action of the RIO.

For vertical rectus muscle palsies the head tilt is not as characteristic. If the yoke oblique muscle overacts, the head tilt may serve to compensate for this overaction rather than to prevent the necessity of the paretic muscle to contract. It is sufficient to remember that the face is often turned to the ipsilateral side to place the eye in the adducted position for both superior and inferior rectus muscle palsies. The chin may be elevated in superior rectus muscle palsies (Fig. 7.60) and depressed in inferior rectus muscle palsies

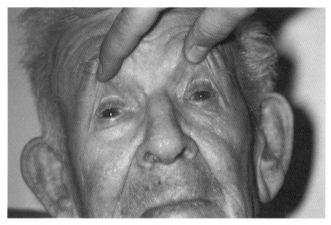

Fig. 7.59: Common head position for a patient with a right inferior oblique muscle palsy. The head is tilted to the same side, the face is turned to the opposite side, and the chin is elevated.

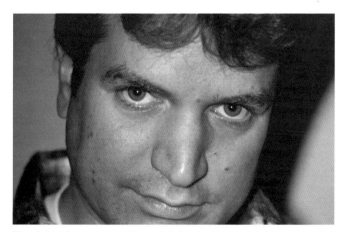

Fig. 7.58: Common head position for a patient with a right superior oblique muscle palsy. The head is tilted and the face is turned to the opposite side, and the chin is depressed.
Source: Catalano RA, Manley DR, Calhoun JH. Measurement of vertical deviations in different gaze positions in patients with a superior oblique palsy. J Ped Ophthalmol and Strabismus. 1988; 25:221.

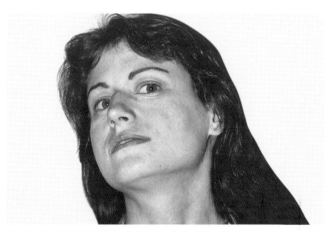

Fig. 7.60: Common head position for a patient with a right superior rectus muscle palsy. The face is turned to the same side and the chin is elevated. This patient also tilts her head to the same side to place the right eye completely out of the field of action of the superior rectus muscle.

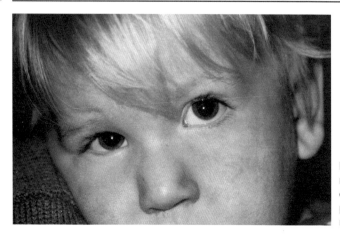

Fig. 7.61: Common head position for a patient with a right inferior rectus muscle palsy. The face is turned to the same side and the chin is depressed. This patient also tilts his head to the same side to place the right eye completely out of the field of action of the inferior rectus muscle.

(Fig. 7.61) to place the eyes out of the position of action of the involved rectus muscles. However, because the head position in patients with paretic vertical rectus muscle palsies varies so greatly, care should be exercised prior to placing too great an emphasis on the head position in patients with these palsies.

REFERENCES

1. Hirschberg J. Über die Messung des Schieldgrades und die Dosierung der Schieloperation, Zentrabl. Prakt Augenheilkd. 1885;8:325.

2. Krimsky E. The binocular examination of the young child. Am J Ophthalmol. 1943; 26:624.

3. Parks MM. Isolated cyclovertical muscle palsy. Arch Ophthalmol. 1958;60:1027-35.

BIBLIOGRAPHY

1. Guyton DL. Clinical assessment of ocular torsion. Am Orthoptic J. 1983;33:7.

2. Parks MM. Alignment. In: Tasman W, Jaeger EA (Eds). Clinical Ophthalmology. Philadelphia: JB Lippincott Co; 2013.

3. von Noorden GK, Campos EC. Binocular vision and ocular motility, 6th edition. St Louis, Mo: CV Mosby; 2002.

8

Esodeviations

■ PSEUDOESOTROPIA

"Pseudoesotropia" is one of the most common conditions for which an ophthalmologist is asked to evaluate infants. It is characterized by the false appearance of esotropia when the visual axes are aligned accurately. The appearance may be caused by a flat, broad nasal bridge; prominent epicanthal folds; or a narrow interpupillary distance. The observer may see less sclera nasally than would be expected, which creates the impression that the eye is turned in toward the nose, especially when the patient gazes to either side. Pseudoesotropia can be differentiated from a true manifest deviation by the use of the corneal light reflex and the cover/uncover test when possible.

A patient with pseudoesotropia caused by a wide nasal bridge and epicanthal folds is shown in Figure 8.1. Note that the light reflex is centered in each pupil. Figures 8.2A and B show another child with pseudoesotropia. When the epicanthal folds are retracted a more symmetric appearance of the nasal sclera can be observed.

■ CONGENITAL ESOTROPIA

The term "congenital esotropia" is generally understood as describing an esodeviation with an onset prior to 6 months of age. It represents the most common type of strabismus, although its pathogenesis remains uncertain. A history of strabismus in the parents or siblings of affected patients is common.

Ophthalmic Manifestations

Ophthalmic manifestations of congenital esotropia include:
- Large esodeviations of 50 or more prism diopters (deviations of less than 50 prism diopters are less common)

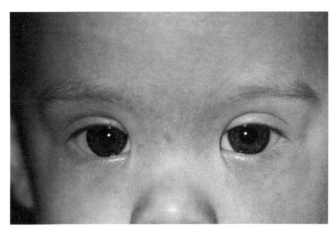

Fig. 8.1: Pseudoesotropia. Note that there is apparently less sclera nasally of the right eye caused by the wide nasal bridge and epicanthal folds.

- Distribution of refractive errors similar to those found in the general population
- Cross-fixation on side gaze and alternation of fixation in primary position
- Amblyopia may develop
- Rotary or latent nystagmus.

A patient with congenital esotropia in the primary position is shown in Figures 8.3A to C. Note the large esodeviation (Fig. 8.3A), cross-fixation with the child using the right eye to gaze left (Fig. 8.3B), and cross-fixation with the child using the left eye to gaze right (Fig. 8.3C).

A child with large-angle congenital esotropia and the modified Krimsky method, in which two base-out prisms are placed apex to apex to measure the esodeviation, is shown in Figures 8.4A and B.

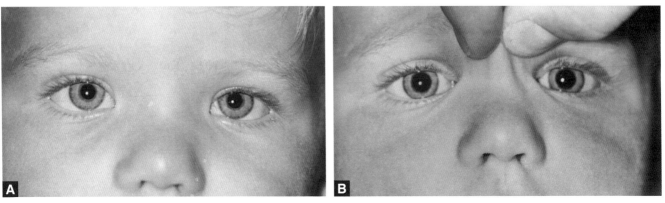

Figs 8.2A and B: Young Child with Pseudotropia. More nasal sclera is noted when the epicanthal fold is retracted.

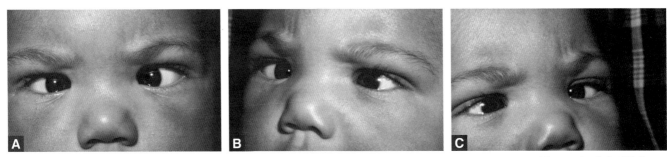

Figs 8.3A to C: (A) Congenital esotropia with a large esodeviation; (B) Cross-fixation with the right eye looking to the left; (C) Cross fixation with the left eye looking to the right.
Source: Nelson LB, Brown GC, Arentson JJ. Recognizing patterns of ocular childhood diseases. Thorofare, NJ: Slack, Inc; 1985.

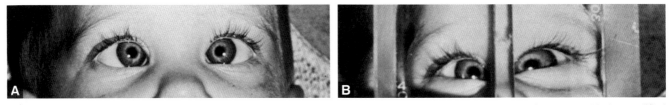

Figs 8.4A and B: (A) Congenital esotropia with a large and constant esotropia; (B) Measuring the amount of estropia with the modified Krimsky method.
Source: Nelson LB, Wagner RS, Simon JW, et al. Congenital esotropia. Surv Ophthalmol. 1987;31:363.

Differential Diagnosis

During the first year of life, a number of conditions can simulate congenital esotropia and cause diagnostic difficulty (Box 8.1). Because the management of these conditions may differ from the treatment of congenital esotropia, their clinical recognition is important.

The diagnosis of congenital esotropia may be confused with congenital sixth nerve palsy. Two diagnostic maneuvers can help distinguish these two conditions. One method of producing abduction in the crossfixating congenital

Box 8.1: Differential diagnosis of congenital esotropia
- Pseudoesotropia
- Duane's retraction syndrome
- Möbius syndrome
- Nystagmus blockage syndrome
- Congenital sixth nerve palsy
- Early onset accommodative esotropia
- Sensory esotropia
- Esotropia in the neurologically impaired

esotrope is to occlude one eye for a short period of time, after which the examiner may note abduction of the uncovered eye. The other method is the doll's head maneuver, in which the examiner turns the child's head in one direction and the eyes shift in the opposite direction.

In a child with congenital esotropia (Figs 8.5A to C) after patching the left eye or performing a doll's head maneuver good abduction can be demonstrated. A child with an inability to abduct the right eye because of a scleral buckle and encircling band from retinal detachment surgery is shown in Figures 8.5D to F. Note the inability to abduct this eye with patching or a doll's head maneuver.

Associated Findings in Congenital Esotropia

Dissociated Vertical Deviation (DVD)

"Dissociated vertical deviation" (DVD) is a slow, upward deviation of one eye or alternate eyes. It may be latent, detected only when the involved eye is covered, or manifest, occurring intermittently or constantly. Occasionally, excyclotorsion can be demonstrated on upward drifting of the eye and incyclotorsion on downward movement. Dissociated vertical deviation can be estimated with Hirschberg's and Krimsky's methods or the prism and cover test. A base-down prism is placed over the involved eye. The strength of the prism is adjusted until no

movement occurs as the cover is shifted from the involved to the fixating eye. Because prism and cover measurement is difficult and can be inaccurate, some observers prefer to estimate DVD on a semiquantitive grading (1 to 4 +).

Inferior Oblique Overaction (IOOA)

"Inferior oblique overaction" (IOOA) results in elevation of the involved eye as it moves into its field of action. It can be classified as grade I through grade IV. Grade I represents 1 mm of higher elevation of the adducting eye in upward gaze. Grade IV indicates 4 mm of higher elevation. These differences in elevation between the two eyes are measured from the 6 o'clock positions on each limbus.

Both DVD and IOOA can cause excessive elevation of one or both eyes in adduction in patients with congenital esotropia. The differentiating features of these two conditions are listed in Table 8.1.

A child with DVD of the right eye is shown in Figures 8.6A to I. Note that when the right eye is covered in the abducting (Figs 8.6A to C), primary (Figs 8.6D to F), or adducting (Figs 8.6G to I) positions it elevates. This is seen after the cover is removed.

Figures 8.7A to C show a patient with overaction of the right inferior oblique muscle. When the left eye is covered the right eye comes down to take up fixation. When the left eye cover is removed the right eye elevates again. Note the absence of elevation of the left eye in the

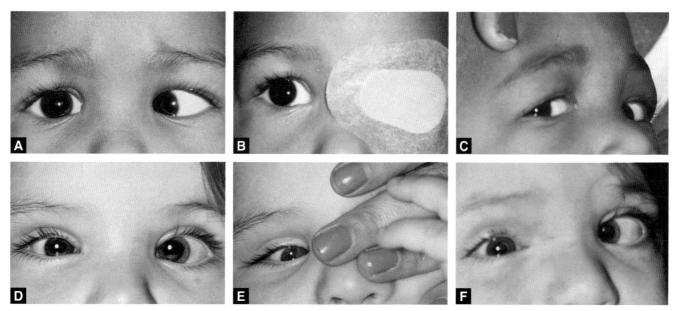

Figs 8.5A to F: (A) A child with congenital esotropia; (B) When patching the left eye, the right eye abducts; (C) Doll's head maneuver demonstrates full abduction of the right eye; (D) A child with retinopathy of prematurity who has a buckle following retinal detachment surgery; (E) Occluding left eye, no abduction of the right eye; (F) Doll's head maneuver demonstrates inability to abduct the right eye because of the restriction from the buckle.

Table 8.1: Distinguishing features of DVD and IOOA*

DVD	IOOA
• Causes elevation in adduction and abduction	• Causes elevation in adduction, not abduction
• Usually comitant, i.e. same in adduction, primary position and abduction	• Incomitant, more in field of action of inferior oblique
• Variability of hyperdeviation	• Not variable
• Usually not associated with an A or a V pattern	• Commonly associated with a V pattern
• Same amount of hyperdeviation in upward gaze and downward gaze	• More hypertropia in upward gaze than downward gaze
• Hyperdeviation may be associated with torsional movement and abduction	• Hyperdeviation not associated with torsional movement
• No corresponding hypotropia in opposite eye	• Corresponding hypotropia in opposite eye

*DVD: Dissociated vertical deviation; IOOA: Inferior oblique overaction.
Source: Modified from Scott WE, Sutton VJ, Thalacker JA. Superior rectus recessions for dissociated vertical deviation. Ophthalmology. 1982;89:317.

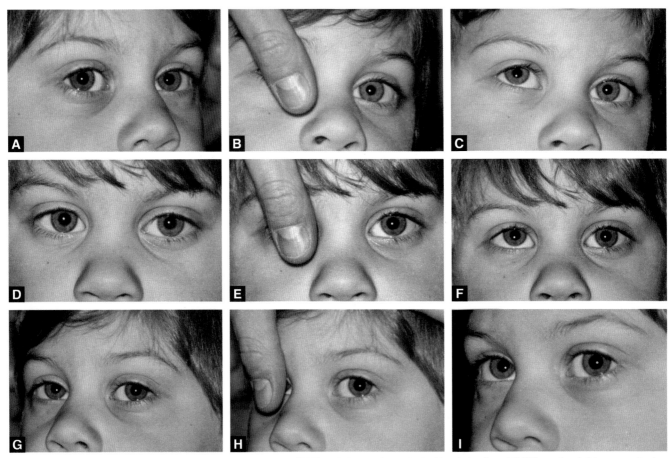

Figs 8.6A to I: (A) A child who has a DVD of the right eye; (B) The right eye is occluded in abduction; (C) When the right eye occlusion is removed, the eye is elevated; (D) The child with a right DVD; (E) The right eye is occluded in the primary position; (F) Note when the right eye occlusion is removed, it is elevated; (G) The child with a right DVD; (H) The right eye is occluded in the adducting position; (I) Note when the right eye occlusion is removed, it is elevated.

abducting position even when a cover is placed over the eye and removed. When the patient is in primary position with a cover placed over the right eye, elevation of that eye did not occur behind the cover (Figs 8.7D to F).

With the patient gazing right, there is no overaction of the left inferior oblique muscle (Figs 8.7G to I). Note that when the right eye is covered, that eye did not elevate behind the cover.

NYSTAGMUS BLOCKAGE SYNDROME

The nystagmus blockage syndrome (NBS) is characterized by nystagmus that begins in infancy and is associated with esotropia. The nystagmus is reduced or absent with the fixating eye in adduction. As the fixating eye follows a target moving laterally toward the primary position and then into abduction, the nystagmus increases and the esotropia decreases. A face turn develops in the direction of the uncovered eye when the fellow eye is occluded. This abnormal head posture allows the uncovered eye to remain in an adducted position. When a base-out prism is placed before the fixating eye the fellow eye will remain in adduction, and the esotropia will actually increase. Figures 8.8A to C show a child with NBS and esotropia in the primary position. Note that when either eye is covered the child will turn her face in the direction of the uncovered eye in order to maintain that eye in the adducting position.

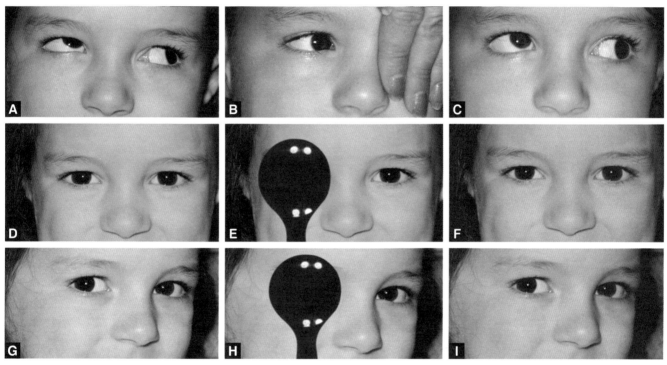

Figs 8.7A to I: (A) Overaction of the inferior oblique muscle. When the left is covered (B), the right eye comes into a position of fixation. When the cover is removed, the right eye elevates again (C). No vertical deviation in primary position (D). (E) Occlusion of the right eye in primary position. No vertical deviation of the right eye when the occluded is removed in primary position (F); (G) No vertical deviation of the right eye in abduction; (H) Occlusion of the right eye in abduction, no elevation of the right eye when the occluded is removed (I).

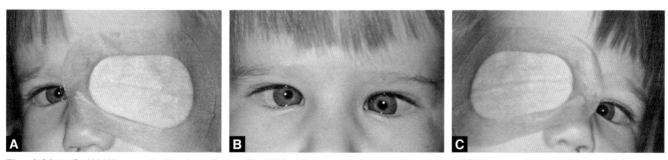

Figs 8.8A to C: (A) When occluding the left eye of a child with congenital esotropia and the NBS, she turns her head to the right to place the uncovered eye in the adducting position; (B) Large esotropia in the primary position; (C) When occluding the right eye of a child with the NBS, she turns her head to the left to place the uncovered eye in the adducting position.

■ ACQUIRED COMITANT ESODEVIATIONS

Accommodative Esotropia

"Accommodative esotropia" is defined as a convergent deviation of the eyes associated with activation of the accommodative reflex. Two types of accommodative esodeviation occur; one is referred to as refractive and is associated with a normal accommodative convergence to accommodation (AC/A) ratio, and the other is termed nonrefractive and is associated with a high AC/A ratio (see Chapter 7).

Ophthalmic Manifestations: For both types of accommodative esodeviations, the following ophthalmic manifestations occur:

- Acquired esotropia with onset from 6 months of age to 7 years (average 2.5 years of age)
- Intermittency of the deviation for a variable period from onset
- Amblyopia common
- Usually no symptoms of diplopia because a facultative suppression scotoma develops in deviating eye
- Both types may occur in the same patient.

Refractive Accommodative Esotropia

In refractive accommodative esotropia (normal AC/A ratio) high hyperopia averaging +4.75 diopters occurs. The deviation is the same for distant and near fixation. The angle of deviation is usually less than 30 prism diopters.

Two children with moderate angles of esotropia are shown in Figures 8.9 and 8.10. With the appropriate hyperopic spectacles the esotropia is reduced.

Nonrefractive Accommodative Esotropia

In nonrefractive accommodative esotropia (high AC/A ratio) refractive errors are normal for age, averaging + 2.25 diopters. When this condition occurs in the absence of refractive accommodative esotropia, typically little or no deviation occurs at distant fixation, but esotropia occurs at near fixation. Esotropia may occur at near fixation only when the patient is fixating small accommodative targets (see Fig. 7.8).

Figures 8.11A to D show a child who has both a refractive and a nonrefractive accommodative esotropia. With hyperopic spectacles at far fixation, no esotropia is noted. When the child fixates a near accommodative target, esotropia is again apparent. The latter is the nonrefractive component. This near esotropia is reduced when the patient looks through bifocals.

Partial or Decompensated Accommodative Esotropia

Refractive or nonrefractive accommodative esotropias do not always occur in their "pure" forms. Affected patients may have a significant reduction in their esodeviation when wearing glasses with or without bifocals. However, if a residual esodeviation persists in spite of full hyperopic correction, deteriorated or nonaccommodative esotropia exists. This condition will more likely occur when the esotropia first presents prior to 1 year of age, when there is a delay of months between the onset of accommodative esotropia and the institution of anti-accommodative therapy, or when there is a severely high AC/A ratio. A child with an esotropia that is not altered by wearing the appropriate hyperopic glasses is shown in Figures 8.12A and B.

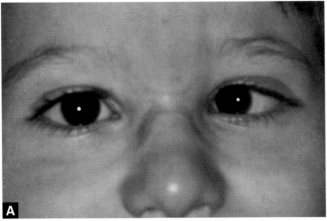 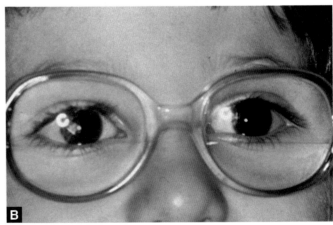

Figs 8.9A and B: (A) A child with accommodative esotropia with out glasses demonstrating a moderate esotropia; (B) The eyes are orthophonic with hyperopic glasses on.

Nonaccommodative Acquired Esotropia

"Spasm of the near synkinetic reflex" is characterized by intermittent episodes of sustained maximal convergence with accommodative spasm and miosis (Figs 8.13A and B). Spasm of the near synkinetic reflex (Fig. 8.14A) even with occluding the left eye, the right eye sustained convergence (Fig. 8.14B). "Sensory deprivation esodeviation" may result from any cause of reduced visual acuity in one eye. Figure 8.15 shows a patient with a cataract and poor vision in the left eye, who presents with a left esotropia.

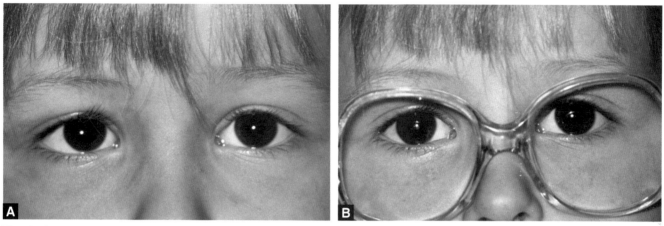

Figs 8.10A and B: (A) Moderate angle esotropia; (B) The eyes are straight with hyperopic glasses on.

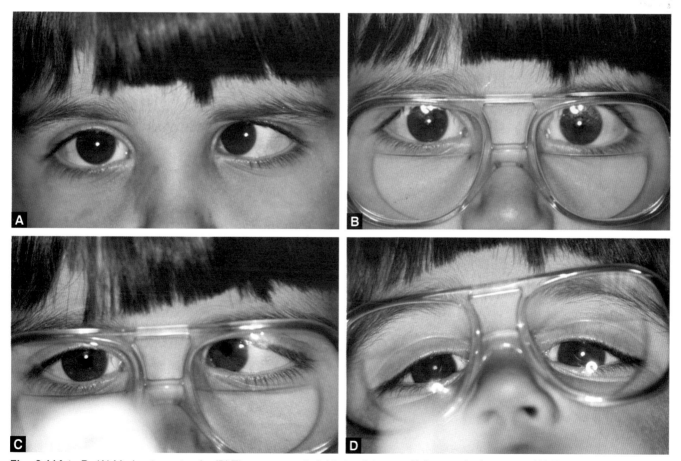

Figs 8.11A to D: (A) Moderate esotropia; (B) The eyes are straight at a distance with hyperopic glasses on; (C) Note the esotropia when fixating on a nearby object; (D) The eyes are straight when focusing on a nearby object through the bifocal.

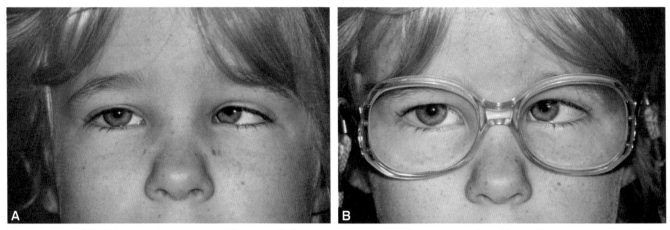

Figs 8.12A and B: (A) Moderate esotropia; (B) Even with the appropriate hyperopic correction, the child continues to have esotropia.

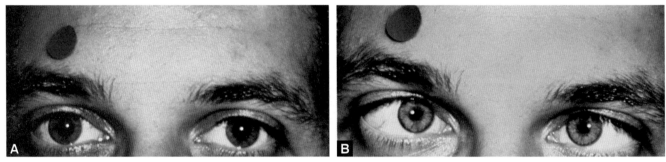

Figs 8.13A and B: (A) Spasm of the near synkinetic reflex. Eyes are initially straight; (B) Sustained maximal convergence with accommodate spasm and miosis.

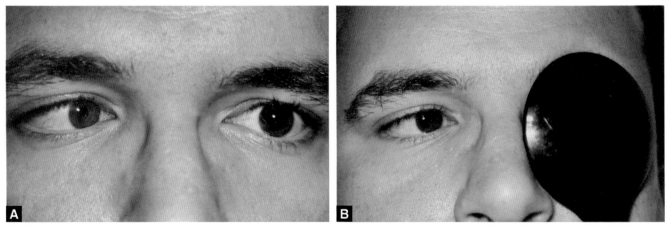

Figs 8.14A and B: (A) Accommodative spasm; (B) Even when the left eye is occluded, the right eye maintained a convergent position.

"Stress-induced esodeviation" may be precipitated by emotional trauma, debilitating illness, physical injury, or aging. "Divergence insufficiency" is characterized by an esodeviation greater at distant fixation than at near fixation. Fusional divergence is reduced. There are no associated neurologic abnormalities. "Divergence paralysis" is characterized by the same ophthalmic findings as those in divergence insufficiency except that it occurs in association with pontine tumors, head trauma, or other neurologic conditions. "Cyclic esotropia" is discussed in Chapter 13.

■ ACQUIRED INCOMITANT ESODEVIATION

Medial Rectus Restriction

An "excessively resected medial rectus muscle" may result in an abduction deficit with increasing esotropia in gaze away from the affected eye. A "medial orbital wall fracture" may be isolated or associated with orbital floor fractures (see Chapter 13) or roof fractures. The nasal orbital contents, including the medial rectus, may become incarcerated within the fracture of the laminae papyracea. This results in restriction of the horizontal ocular movements.

A patient with a left medial wall fracture with significant restriction to abduction of the left eye, causing an incomitant esotropia (Fig. 8.16A). Patient was able to adduct left eye normally (Fig. 8.16B).

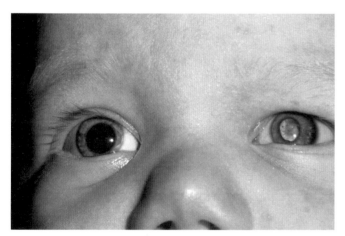

Fig. 8.15: Dense cataract in the left eye resulted in poor vision and a sensory esotropia.

A patient with a left medial orbital wall fracture that resulted in the inability to abduct the left eye even to the midline is shown in Figure 8.17. A computed tomogram shows the left medial orbital wall fracture (Fig. 8.18).

"Thyroid myopathy" (see Chapter 13) causes pathologic changes in the extraocular muscles, resulting in restricted eye movements. Figures 8.19A to C show a patient with thyroid myopathy with an esotropia. Note the inability to abduct the left eye even to the midline. The abduction deficit results in an incomitant esotropia.

Lateral Rectus Weakness

"Sixth nerve palsy" causes an esotropia in the primary position, which increases in the field of action of the paretic lateral rectus muscle. The palsy may be unilateral or bilateral. Continuation of binocular vision is usually possible by maintenance of both eyes in the gaze position away from the palsied eye; this results in a compensatory horizontal face turn toward the eye with the palsied muscle.

Figures 8.20A to D show a congenital left sixth nerve palsy in an otherwise healthy child, demonstrating an incomitant esotropia. A left face turn achieves orthophoria (Fig. 8.20A). With the head positioned straight a left esotropia is manifest (Fig. 8.20B). Gaze to the left demonstrates no abduction of the left eye past the midline (Fig. 8.20C). Gaze to the right is normal (Fig. 8.20D). A child with an intracranial tumor who developed bilateral asymmetric sixth nerve palsy is shown in Figures 8.21A to C. Note that the greatest esotropia is in right gaze.

A "slipped" or "lost lateral rectus muscle" causes esotropia of the involved eye. The esotropia is worse in gaze toward the involved eye. Figures 8.22A and B show a

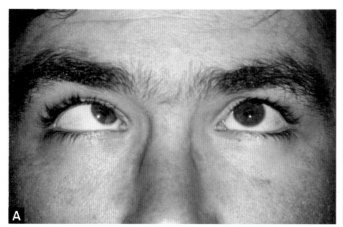
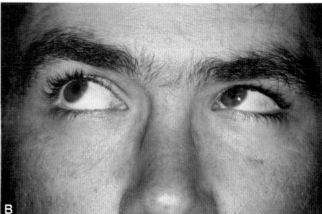

Figs 8.16A and B: (A) Left medial wall fracture with inability to abduct left eye; (B) Adduction of the left eye was normal.

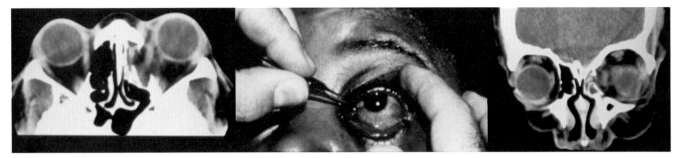

Fig. 8.17: Left medial wall fracture with an inability to abduct the eye even with forced ductions.

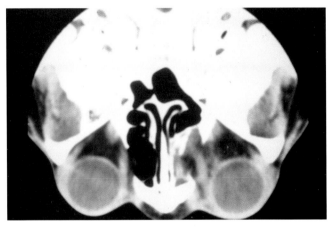

Fig. 8.18: A computed tomogram demonstrates the left medial wall fracture from the patient in Figure 8.17.

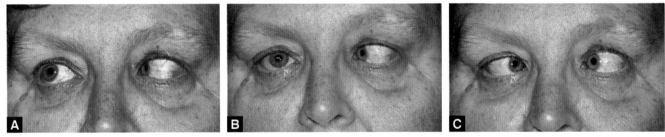

Figs 8.19A to C: (A) Thyroid ophthalmyopathy with normal gaze right; (B) Primary position large esotropia; (C) Inability to abduct left eye.

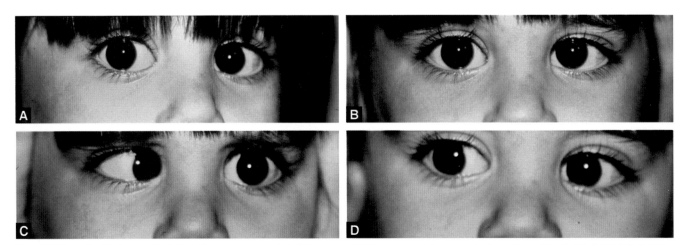

Figs 8.20A to D: (A) Congenital left sixth nerve palsy with left face turn; (B) Head straight demonstrates left esotropia; (C) Gaze left demonstrates no abduction past the midline; (D) Gaze right showing no narrowing of the palpebral fissure usually noted in Duane syndrome.
Source: Nelson LB, Wagner RS, Simon JW, et al. Congenital esotropia. Surv Ophthalmol. 1987;31:363.

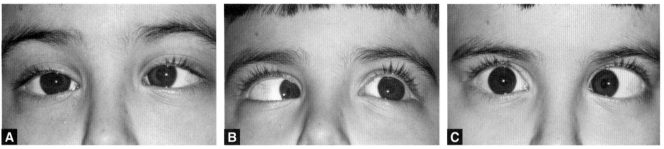

Figs 8.21A to C: (A) Bilateral asymmetric sixth nerve palsy in primary position; (B) Left gaze with decrease abduction; (C) Right gaze inability to abduct beyond the midline.

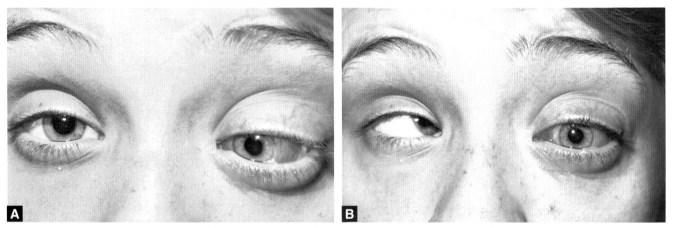

Figs 8.22A and B: (A) Large esotropia following retinal detachment surgery to the left eye; (B) Slipped left lateral rectus muscle with inability to abduct left eye.
Source: Hiller TL, Nelson LB, Brown GC, et al. The sliped rectus muscle. Ophthalmic Surg. 1985;16:315.

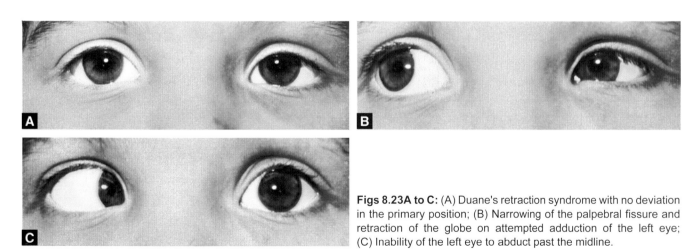

Figs 8.23A to C: (A) Duane's retraction syndrome with no deviation in the primary position; (B) Narrowing of the palpebral fissure and retraction of the globe on attempted adduction of the left eye; (C) Inability of the left eye to abduct past the midline.

patient who underwent a retinal detachment repair, and a left medial rectus recession and lateral rectus resection for a sensory esotropia. Postoperatively, her explant eroded into the lateral rectus insertion, detaching the muscle from the globe. The left lateral rectus was discovered attached to the sclera, 10 mm from the original insertion. Note the

left esotropia in the primary position with an inability to abduct the left eye.

"Type I Duane's retraction syndrome" (DRS) (see Chapter 13) results in severe limitation of abduction of the involved eye (Figs 8.23A to C). Note the large esotropia in left gaze.

■ BIBLIOGRAPHY

1. Mohney BG. Common forms of childhood esotropia. Ophthalmol. 2001;108:805.
2. Nelson LB, Wagner RS, Simon JW, et al. Congenital esotropia. Surv Ophthamol. 1987;31:363.
3. Preslan MW, Beauchamp GR. Accommodative esotropia: Review of current practices and controversies. Ophthalmic Surg. 1987;18:68.
4. Raab EL. Etiologic factors in accommodative esodeviation. Trans Am Ophthalmol Soc. 1982;80:657.
5. von Noorden GK. A reassessment of infantile esotropia. XLIV Edward Jackson Memorial Lecture . Am J Ophthalmol. 1988;105:1.

Exodeviations

◼ PSEUDOEXOTROPIA

"Pseudoexotropia" may occur in the presence of a positive angle kappa (see Figs 7.16A to C) or a wide interpupillary distance. A child with pseudoexotropia is shown in Figures 9.1A to C. Note that when either eye is covered the uncovered eye maintains its "straight ahead" position. Figures 9.2A to I show pseudoexotropia caused by retinopathy of prematurity and dragged maculas of both eyes in a child who is highly myopic. Covering the eye that is directed straight ahead demonstrates that the patient is fixating with his pseudoexotropic eye. Note the straightening of the posterior pole vessels and ectopic maculas.

◼ CONGENITAL EXOTROPIA

Exotropia occurring before the age of 1 year in an otherwise healthy child is rare. Although "congenital exotropia" may go through a period of intermittency, many cases progress quickly to a constant alternating exotropia. The angle of deviation is often large, averaging 35 prism diopters or greater. Figures 9.3A and B show large-angle exotropia in a child younger than 1 year of age. Figure 9.4 shows congenital exotropia in a child who alternates freely.

◼ ACQUIRED COMITANT EXODEVIATIONS

"Exophoria" is a divergent deviation that is kept latent by sensory fusion (see Fig. 7.1).

"Intermittent exotropia" is the most common divergent strabismus in childhood. The age of onset varies but is often between 6 months and 4 years. Initially, the deviation is usually intermittent and greater at distant fixation; often there is no deviation at near fixation in the early stages. A patient with intermittent exotropia is shown in Figures 9.5A and B. The eyes are straight, but when a cover is placed

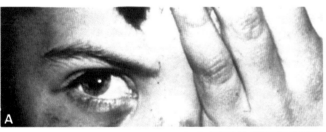

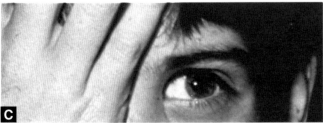

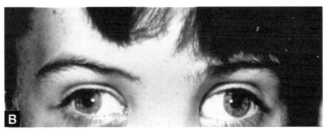

Figs 9.1A to C: Pseudoexotropia. Regardless of whether the left or right is occluded, the eyes maintain its straight ahead position without a refixation movement.

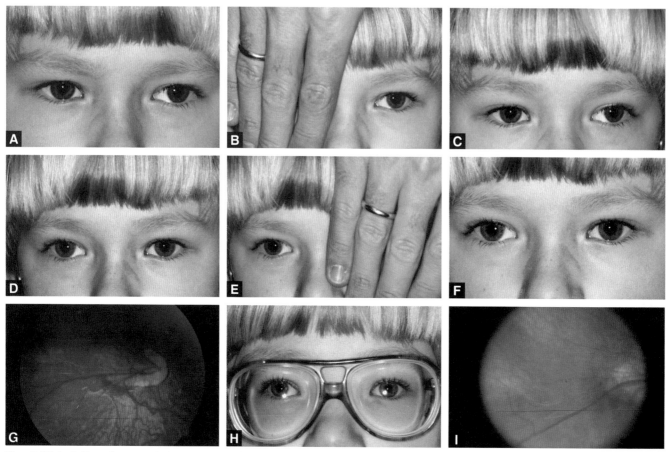

Figs 9.2A to I: Pseudoexotropia in a child caused by retinopathy of prematurity and dragged maculas of both eyes.

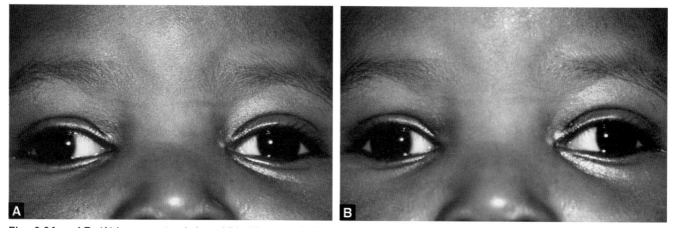

Figs 9.3A and B: (A) Large exotropia in a child with congenital exotropia fixation with the left eye; (B) Fixating with the right eye.

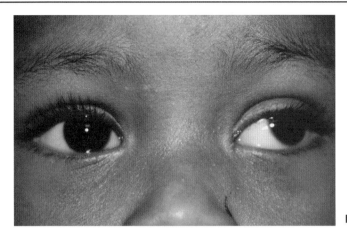

Fig. 9.4: Congenital exotropia.

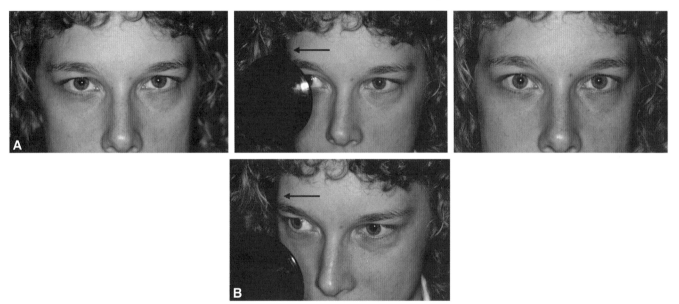

Figs 9.5A and B: Patient with intermittent exotropia. Note that on occlusion, the eye under cover drifts out.

in front of the right eye sensory fusion is interrupted, and the eye drifts out. When the cover is removed, the right eye stays exotropic. Figures 9.6A and B show intermittent exotropia in a patient with good binocular function. The right eye drifts outward temporally only with fatigue, illness, or daydreaming.

"Basic exotropia" in a patient who alternates freely and has equal vision in each eye is shown in Figures 9.7A and B. This patient had intermittent exotropia, which progressed over the years to a constant exotropia. The distance deviation was equal to the near deviation.

"Sensory exotropia" results from unilateral visual impairment from a variety of causes, followed by disruption of fusion. Figure 9.8 shows a patient with severe

anisometropic amblyopia of the left eye (visual acuity 20/400) with a large left exotropia.

"Convergence insufficiency" is characterized by an exodeviation that is greater at near fixation than at distant fixation, associated with asthenopic symptoms for near visual tasks and reduced amplitudes of convergence. Figures 9.9A and B show a patient who was orthophoric for distant fixation, with 12 prism diopters of exophoria at near fixation.

"Consecutive exotropia" occurs either spontaneously in a formerly esotropic patient or iatrogenically after surgery for esotropia. Figures 9.10A and B show a patient with a consecutive alternating exotropia following a bilateral medial rectus recession for esotropia.

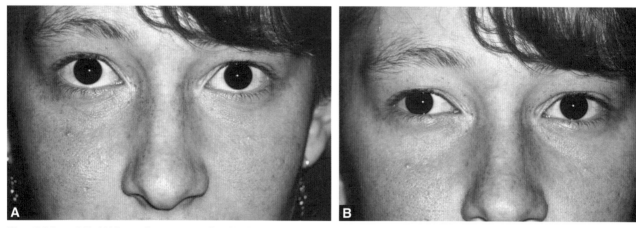

Figs 9.6A and B: (A) Intermittent exotropia with the eyes straight; (B) The right eye drifts out with inattention.

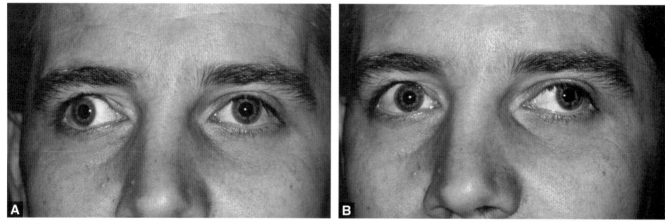

Figs 9.7A and B: (A) Large alternate constant exotropia with the left eye fixating; (B) Now the right eye is fixating.

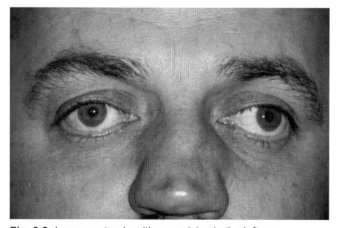

Fig. 9.8: Large exotropia with poor vision in the left eye.

■ ACQUIRED INCOMITANT EXODEVIATIONS

"Third nerve palsy" with an exotropia in the primary position and an inability to adduct the eye causes a greater exotropia in gaze away from the affected eye. Figures 9.11A to E show a child with a right third nerve palsy with an exotropia in primary gaze and ptosis. An inability to depress, elevate, or adduct the right eye occurred in this patient. Note that the greater exotropia is in left gaze. A child with a right third nerve palsy with a large right exotropia is shown in Figures 9.12A to C. The right eye was not able to adduct, even to the midline, causing a greater exotropia in left gaze.

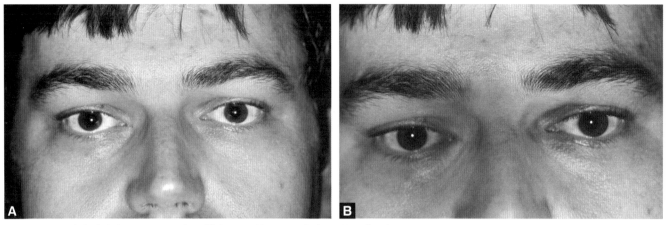

Figs 9.9A and B: (A) Convergence insufficiency with no deviation when fixating at a distance; (B) Divergent deviation on fixating at a near target.

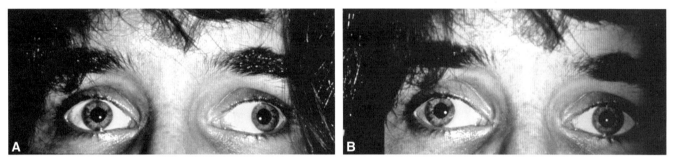

Figs 9.10A and B: (A) Consecutive exotropia with the right eye fixating; (B) Left eye fixating and the right eye deviated outward.

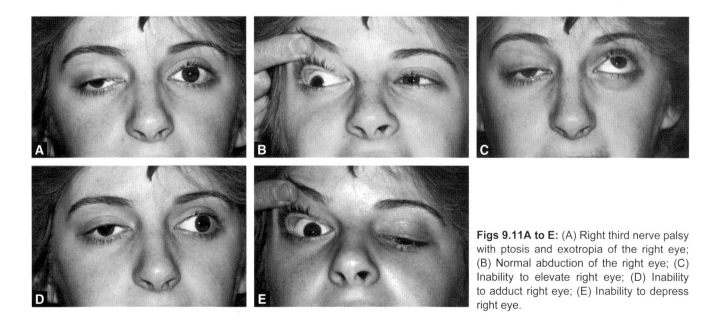

Figs 9.11A to E: (A) Right third nerve palsy with ptosis and exotropia of the right eye; (B) Normal abduction of the right eye; (C) Inability to elevate right eye; (D) Inability to adduct right eye; (E) Inability to depress right eye.

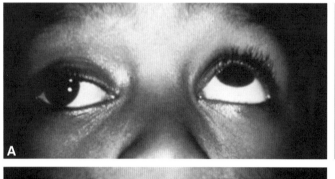

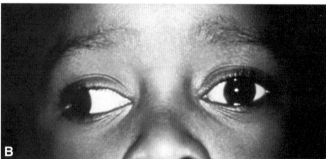

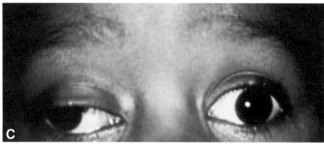

Figs 9.12A to C: (A) Right third nerve palsy with an inability for the right eye to elevate; (B) In primary position large right exotropia; (C) No movement of the right in adduction with ptosis (aberrant regeneration).
Photo Courtesy: Robison D Harley.
Source: Nelson LB. Pediatric Ophthalmology. Philadelphia: WB Saunders Co; 1984.

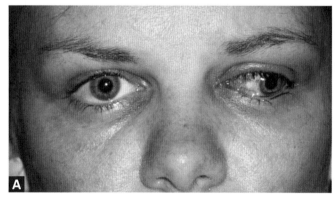

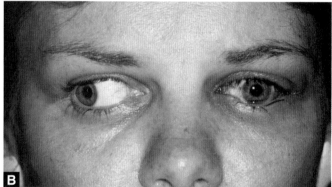

Figs 9.13A and B: (A) Slipped left medial rectus muscle with large exotropia in primary positions; (B) Inability to adduct left eye past the midline.

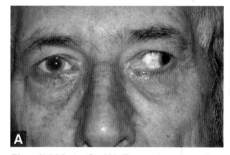

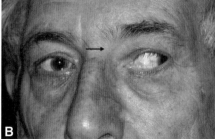

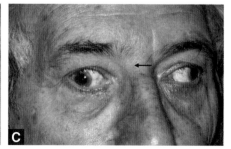

Figs 9.14A to C: (A) Excessive resection of the left lateral rectus demonstrating a large exotropia in primary position; (B) Normal abduction of the left eye; (C) Inability to adduct the left even to the midline.

A "slipped" or "lost medial rectus" results in an exotropia with a greater exodeviation in gaze away from the affected eye. A patient who had undergone an 8-mm resection of the left medial rectus and an 8-mm recession of the left lateral rectus four days earlier is shown in Figures 9.13A and B. Note the large exotropia in the primary position, which increases in right gaze, and the inability to adduct the left eye.

"Excessive resection" of the lateral rectus can result in an incomitant exotropia (Figs 9.14A to C). Note the large exotropia in the primary position and the inability to adduct the left eye past the midline.

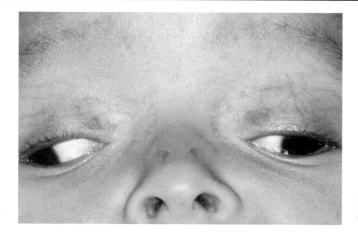

Fig. 9.15: Generalized fibrosis syndrome with ptosis and large exotropia.

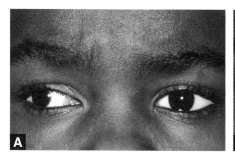 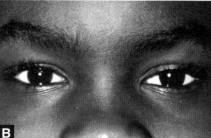 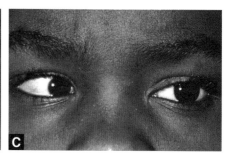

Figs 9.16A to C: (A) Type II DRS of the left eye with decrease adduction of the left eye and a large exotropia; (B) In primary position mild left exotropia; (C) Decrease abduction of the left eye.

"Tight lateral rectus muscles", which may be part of the generalized fibrosis syndrome (see Chapter 13), result in a large exotropia. Figure 9.15 shows a 2-month-old child with severe ptosis and an exotropia greater than 100 prism diopters. During surgery, the lateral recti were fibrotic, with a positive forced-duction test to adduction.

"Type II Duane's retraction syndrome" (DRS) (see Chapter 13) is characterized by restricted adduction and slightly limited or normal abduction. Exotropia increases in gaze away from the involved eye (Figs 9.16A to C). Note the large exotropia in right gaze in type II DRS of the left eye.

■ BIBLIOGRAPHY

1. Burke MJ. Intermittent exotropia. In: Nelson LB, Wagner RS (Eds). Strabismus Surgery. Boston: Little, Brown & Co;1985.
2. Govindan M, Mohney BG, Diehl NN, et al. Incidence and types of childhood exotropia: a population-based study. Ophthalmol. 2005;112:104.
3. Hermann JS. Surgical therapy for convergence insufficiency. J Pediatr Ophthalmol Strabismus. 1981;18:28.
4. `Richard JM, Parks MM. Intermittent exotropia: surgical results in different age groups. Ophthalmol. 1983;90:1172.
5. Rubin SE, Nelson LB, Wagner RS, et al. Infantile exotropia in healthy children. Ophthalmic Surg. 1988;19:792.
6. Scott WE, Keech R, Mash AJ. The postoperative results and stability of exodeviations. Arch Ophthalmol. 1981;99:1814.

10

A and V Patterns

■ INTRODUCTION

"A" and "V" patterns are manifested by a horizontal change of alignment as the eyes move from the primary position to midline upward gaze and downward gaze. These patterns are demonstrated by measuring a deviation in the primary position and with the eyes directed approximately 25° in upward gaze and downward gaze while the patient fixates on a distant object. Between upward gaze and downward gaze, a difference of 10 prism diopters in the horizontal alignment is usually sufficient to diagnose an "A" pattern, and a difference of 15 prism diopters diagnoses a "V" pattern.

■ "A" PATTERN IN ESOTROPIA

Esotropia increases in straight upward gaze and decreases in straight downward gaze (Figs 10.1A to C). This child maintained a chin up where the esotropia was least.

Figures 10.2A to C show a patient with a significant esotropia in upward gaze, mild esotropia in primary gaze and no esotropia in downward gaze.

■ "A" PATTERN IN EXOTROPIA

Exotropia increases in straight downward gaze and decreases in straight upward gaze (Figs 10.3A to C). The overaction of both superior oblique muscles causes increased abduction in downward gaze. Underaction of both inferior muscles causes decreased abduction in upward gaze.

■ "V" PATTERN IN ESOTROPIA

Esotropia increases in straight downward gaze and decreases in straight upward gaze (Figs 10.4A to I). Note the overaction of both inferior oblique muscles, which

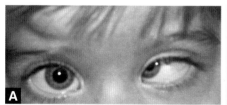
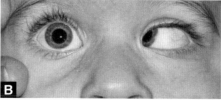
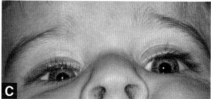

Figs 10.1A to C: (A) A-pattern esotropia with large esotropia in up-gaze; (B) Large esotropia in primary position; (C) Minimal esotropia in down-gaze.

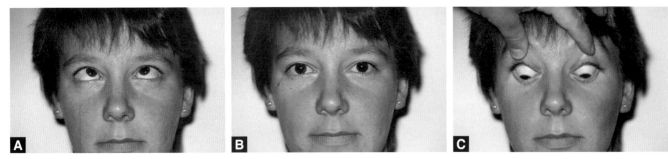

Figs 10.2A to C: (A) A-pattern esotropia with a large esotropia in up-gaze; (B) Mild esotropia in primary position; (C) Orthophoric in down-gaze.

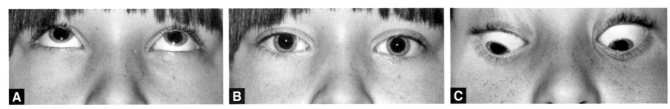

Figs 10.3A to C: (A) A-pattern exotropia with mild exotropia in up-gaze; (B) Slightly larger exotropia in primary position; (C) Large exotropia in down-gaze.

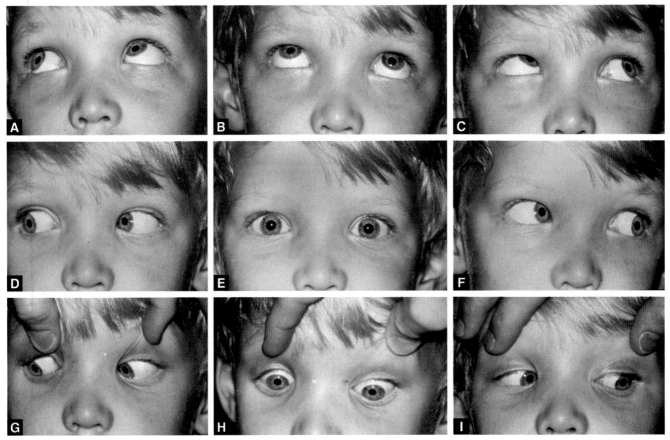

Figs 10.4A to I: V-pattern esotropia with less esotropia in up-gaze than in down-gaze (B and H). Mild esotropia in primary position (E). Note the overaction of the inferior oblique muscles (A and C). Even in side-gaze, the eye in adduction is elevated compared to the abducting eye (D and F). Note the underaction of the superior oblique muscles (G and I).

causes increased abduction in upward gaze. Underaction of both superior oblique muscles causes decreased abduction in downward gaze. "V" pattern esotropia in a patient with a significant esotropia in straight downward gaze which decreases in primary position, although it is still quite large (Figs 10.5A to C). In straight upward gaze the esotropia, which is still present, is less.

■ "V" PATTERN IN EXOTROPIA

Exotropia increases in straight upward gaze and decreases in straight downward gaze (Figs 10.6A to I). Figures 10.7A to I show a patient with an overaction of the left inferior oblique, an exotropia that increases in straight upward gaze and decreases in straight downward gaze with an underaction of superior obliques and esotropia.

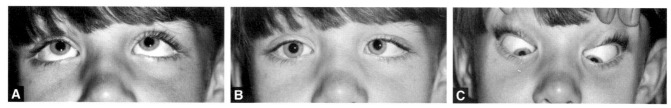

Figs 10.5A to C: V-pattern esotropia. Less esotropia in both up-gaze (A), with moderate esotropia in primary position (B) and greater esotropia in down-gaze (C).

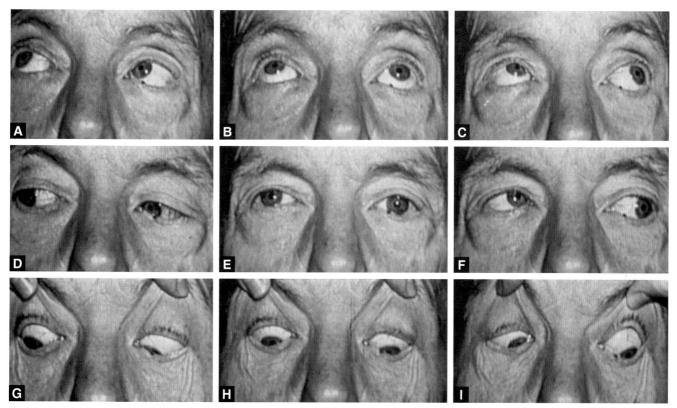

Figs 10.6A to I: Showing a V-pattern exotropia. Note the minimal exotropia in down-gaze (H) with larger exotropia in primary position (E) and a larger exotropia in up-gaze (B). Normal left, inferior oblique (A) but overacting right inferior oblique (C) Elevation of of the right eye in adduction (F) but no elevation of the left eye in adduction (D) slight overaction of the left superior oblique (G) but underaction of the right superior oblique (I).

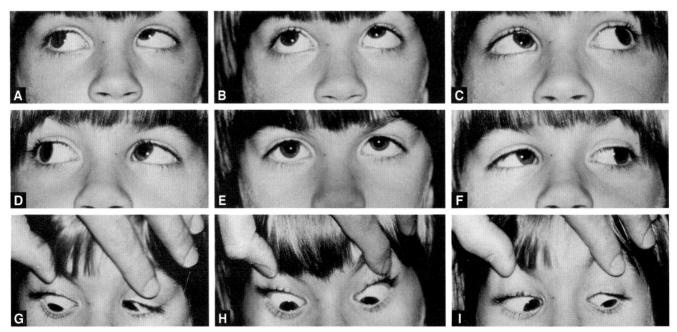

Figs 10.7A to I: Shows a V-pattern exotropia with an esotropia in down-gaze (H) with an exotropia in up-gaze (B). Note the significant overaction of the left inferior oblique muscle (A) and mild overaction of the right inferior oblique muscle (C). Elevations of each eye in adduction (D and F). Underaction of both superior obliques (G and I). Mild exotropia in primary position (E).

■ BIBLIOGRAPHY

1. Breinin GM. Vertically incomitant horizontal strabismus: The A-V patterns. NY State J Med. 1961;61:2243.

2. Knapp P. A and V pattern : Symposium on Strabismus. Trans of the New Orleans Acad Ophthalmol; 1972.

3. Knapp P. Vertically incomitant horizontal strabismus: The so-called A and V syndrome. Trans Am Ophthalmol Soc. 1959;57:666.

Cyclovertical Deviations

■ PSEUDOVERTICAL STRABISMUS

Some children appear to have a vertical deviation when cover testing demonstrates that there is no misalignment of the visual axes. Some of the more common explanations for pseudovertical strabismus include vertical angle kappa, a vertically displaced macula, orbital asymmetry, lid retraction and vertical displacement of the globe by a mass.

A patient with an apparent right hypertropia is shown in Figures 11.1A to C. Note that there is no inferior oblique overaction associated with the patient's pseudohypertropia. Figures 11.2A to C in comparison to Figures 11.1A to C show a patient with a true right hypertropia from a right superior oblique palsy and an overacting right inferior oblique (Figs 11.2A and B). Figures 11.3A and B show a patient with an inferior displacement of the right lower

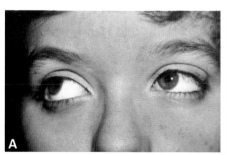
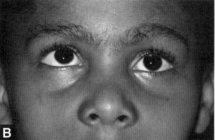
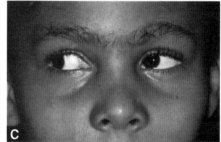

Figs 11.1A to C: Pseudohypertropia of the right eye (B). Note that there is no overaction of the inferior oblique muscles (A and C).

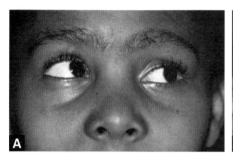
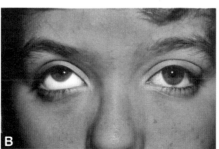
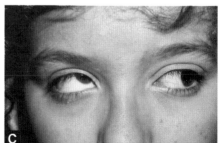

Figs 11.2A to C: Showing a right hypertropia (A and B) due to a right superior oblique palsy with an overacting right inferior oblique muscle (C).

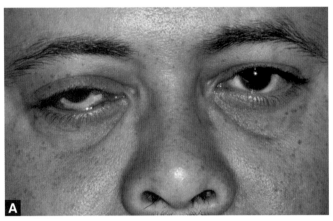
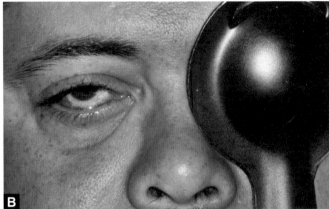

Figs 11.3A and B: (A) Apparent right hypertropia following an inferior rectus recession. Note the sagging of the right lower eyelid; (B) Covering the left eye with no change in the apparent position of the right eye.
Source: Wagner RS, Nelson LB. Complications following strabismus surgery. Int Ophthalmol Clin. 1985;25:171.

eyelid following a 5-mm recession of the right inferior rectus muscle. Note the sagging of the right lower eyelid with apparent right hypertropia. When the left eye is covered, there is no movement of the right eye. A close up of the right lower eyelid sagging is shown in Figure 11.4. The patient had no vertical or oblique muscle dysfunction (Figs 11.5A to F).

OBLIQUE MUSCLE DYSFUNCTIONS

Inferior Oblique Overaction

Inferior oblique overaction (IOOA) may be unilateral or bilateral, and symmetric or asymmetric (see Chapter 8). Inferior oblique overaction results in elevation of the involved eye as it moves nasally. It may occur as an isolated condition or with esotropia or exotropia, often associated with a "V" pattern (see Chapter 10). Because the inferior oblique is an abductor, it will cause more divergence in upward gaze, producing a "V" pattern. Inferior oblique overaction is also commonly found in congenital esotropia (see Chapter 8). Finally, IOOA is frequently observed in superior oblique palsies (discussed later in this chapter).

A child with asymmetric IOOA is shown in Figures 11.6A and B. Note the more significant overacting left inferior oblique. This child had been operated on for congenital esotropia several years earlier.

In the "V" pattern exotropia shown in Figures 11.7A to I, note the overacting inferior obliques and the increased exotropia in upward gaze.

Underaction of the Inferior Oblique

Isolated paresis of the inferior oblique muscle is a rare entity. Patients with an inferior oblique paresis manifest either a hypotropia of the affected eye or a hypertropia

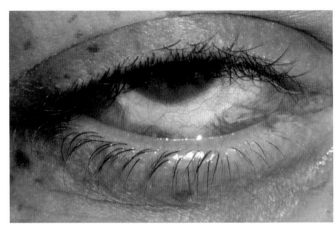

Fig. 11.4: Sagging of the right lower eyelid from Figures 11.3A and B.

of the unaffected eye, depending on fixation preference. The vertical deviation increases on gaze into the field of action of the involved inferior oblique, but decreases in the opposite gaze. Bielschowsky's head-tilting test is positive on tilting the head toward the opposite side. With time, the superior oblique often becomes contracted and shows moderate to marked overaction. Patients typically tilt their heads toward the ipsilateral side in an attempt to decrease the vertical deviation and to maintain binocular vision.

In a patient with left inferior oblique muscle palsy (Figs 11.8A to I), there is a slight left hypotropia in the primary position. Note that the left eye depresses in adduction. Underaction of the left inferior oblique and overaction of the left superior oblique occur.

Superior Oblique Overaction

Superior oblique overaction (SOOA) may be unilateral or bilateral, and symmetric or asymmetric. Occasionally,

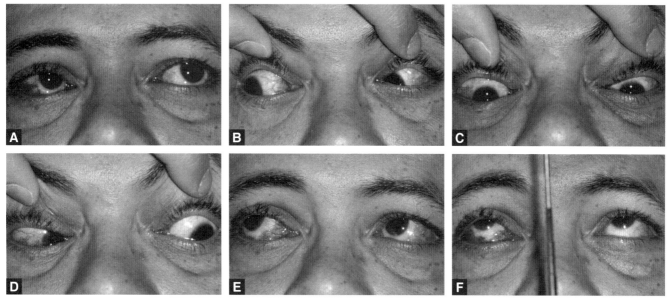

Figs 11.5A to F: Normal inferior oblique function (A and E). Normal elevation and depression (C and F). Normal superior oblique function (B and D). Note that there is no oblique or vertical abnormality from patient in Figures 11.3A and B.

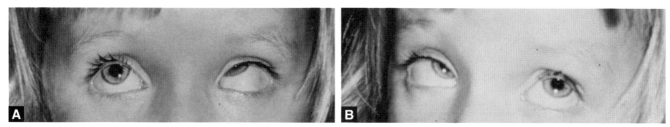

Figs 11.6A and B: Asymmetric overaction of the inferior oblique. The left (A) is greater than the right inferior oblique (B).

SOOA occurs as an isolated condition. However, SOOA is also associated with a horizontal deviation (more frequently with exodeviation than with esodeviation), often with an "A" pattern. Because the superior oblique is an abductor, it will cause more divergence in downward gaze, producing an "A" pattern. Superior oblique overaction is also found in patients with inferior oblique palsies (discussed earlier in this chapter).

A patient with an "A" pattern exotropia with SOOA is shown in Figures 11.9A to C. Note the increased exodeviation in downward gaze. Figures 11.10A to C show a child with SOOA. This child had no horizontal deviation in the primary position.

Underaction of the Superior Oblique

Underaction of the superior oblique (fourth nerve palsy) is the most common cause of an isolated cyclovertical muscle palsy. It can be congenital or acquired. Fourth nerve palsy is initially an incomitant hypertropia, greatest in adducted

depression of the involved eye. If the palsy continues, contracture of the ipsilateral inferior oblique occurs, and the maximum hyperdeviation is found in the field of action of this muscle. Another sign of contracture of the ipsilateral inferior oblique muscle is overelevation of the adducted palsied eye.

Because the superior oblique muscle is a depressor and an intorter, its tone is diminished by upward gaze and by tilting the head to the shoulder opposite the palsied muscle. With the head tilted to the opposite side of the palsied muscle, patients with a unilateral superior oblique palsy can maintain binocular vision (see Fig. 7.58).

Figures 11.11A to I show a young girl with a left superior oblique palsy. Note the left hypertropia, overaction of the left inferior oblique, and underaction of the left superior oblique.

Figures 11.12A to C illustrate that head tilting to the right reduces the left hypertropia, while tilting to the left increases the vertical deviation.

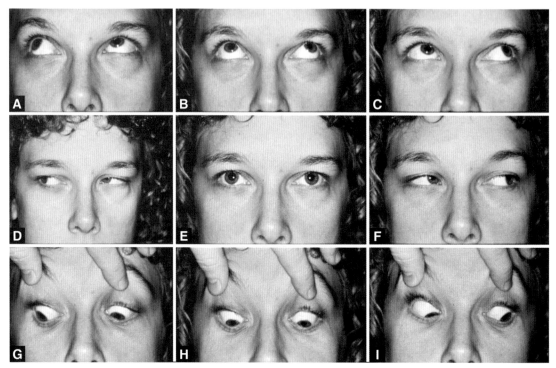

Figs 11.7A to I: V-pattern exotropia with increased exotropia in up-gaze. Note the overacting inferior oblique muscles (A and C). Large exotropia in up-gaze (B) with less exotropia in primary position (E) and minimal exotropia in down-gaze (H). In side-gaze, the adducting eye is elevated (D and F). Mild left superior oblique overaction (G) and moderate overaction of the right superior oblique (I).

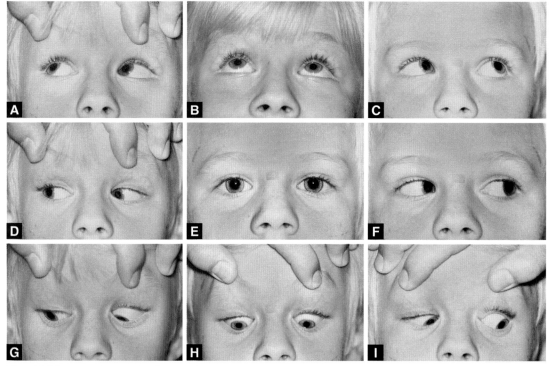

Figs 11.8A to I: Isolated left inferior oblique muscle. Note the underaction of the left inferior oblique (A) and the overaction of the left superior oblique (G). Slight decrease in elevation (B) and depression of the left eye (H). Normal function of the right inferior oblique (C) and superior oblique (I). Left hypotropia in primary (E) and right gaze (D) and orthophoria in left gaze (F).

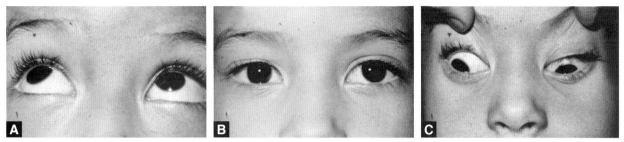

Figs 11.9A to C: Showing A-pattern exotropia with a larger exotropia in down-gaze with overaction of the superior obliques (C) then in primary position (B). There is no exotropia in up-gaze with an underaction of the left inferior oblique (A).

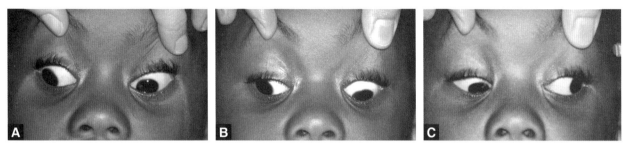

Figs 11.10A to C: Large exotropia in down-gaze (B) due to overaction of the left (A) and the right (C) superior obliques.

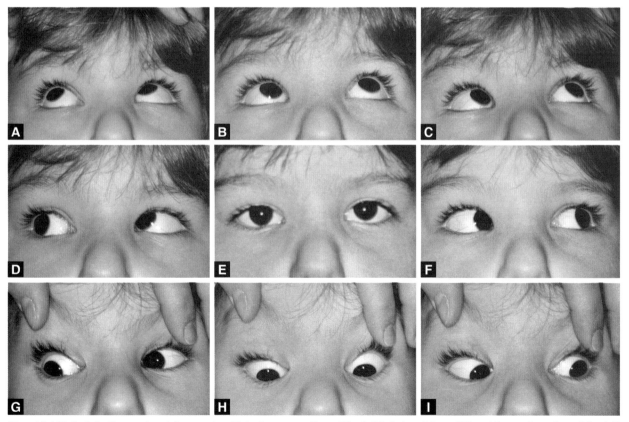

Figs 11.11A to I: Left superior oblique palsy. Note the overaction of the left inferior oblique (A) and the underaction of the left superior oblique (G). Left hypertropia in primary position (E) which increases in right gaze (D) and decreases in left gaze (F). Left hypertropia in up-gaze (B) and down-gaze (H). The right inferior oblique (C) and superior oblique (I) are normal.

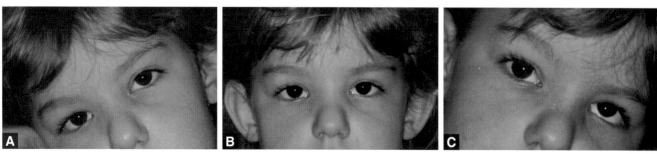

Figs 11.12A to C: Left superior oblique palsy from Figures11.11A to G showing a larger left hypertropia in primary position (B) which increases on tilting to the left (C) compared to tilting to the right (A).

■ BIBLIOGRAPHY

1. Knapp P. Classification and treatment of superior oblique palsy. Am Orthoptic J. 1974;24:18.
2. Mitchell PR, Parks MM. Oblique muscle dysfunctions. In:Tasman W, Jaeger EA (Eds). Clinical Ophthalmology. Philadelphia: JB Lippincott Co; 2013.
3. Parks MM. Isolated cyclovertical muscle palsy. Arch Ophthalmol. 1958;60:1027.
4. Plager DA. Tendon laxity in superior oblique palsy. Ophthalmol. 1992;99:1032.
5. Reese PD, Scott WE. Superior oblique tenotomy in the treatment of isolated inferior oblique paresis. J Pediatr Ophthalmol Strabismus. 1987;24:4.
6. Scott WE, Nankin SJ. Isolated inferior oblique paresis. Arch Ophthalmol. 1977;95:186.

12

Monofixation Syndrome

■ OPHTHALMIC MANIFESTATIONS AND CAUSES

In 1969, Parks[1] defined the monofixation syndrome, in which peripheral fusion and vergence amplitudes capable of maintaining alignment within approximately 10 prism diopters exists despite deficient stereopsis and a central suppression scotoma in one eye, during binocular viewing. Ophthalmic manifestations of the monofixation syndrome are described in Box 12.1. The causes of the monofixation syndrome are listed in Box 12.2.

Box 12.1: Ophthalmic manifestations of the monofixation syndrome

- Horizontal deviation is less than 10 prism diopters
- Macular scotoma in nonfixating eye occurs under binocular conditions
- Peripheral normal retinal correspondence with good fusional vergence amplitudes occurs
- Alternate cover test measurement (latent deviation) may be greater than that of simultaneous prism and cover test
- Stereoacuity is 67–300 seconds of arc
- Amblyopia may occur.

Box 12.2: Causes of the monofixation syndrome

- Primary monofixation syndrome
- Anisometropia
- Strabismus surgery (surgery for esotropia more commonly than surgery for exotropia)
- Organic macular lesion

■ DIAGNOSIS

In order to diagnose the monofixation syndrome, a macular scotoma under binocular conditions with peripheral fusion and fusional vergence amplitudes must be demonstrated. The simultaneous prism and cover test identifies a horizontal deviation of less than 10 prism diopters (see Figs 7.33A to I). A variety of tests can be used to test stereoacuity (see Chapter 4). Horizontal fusional vergence amplitudes are demonstrated by having the patient look through a prism bar or rotary prism. Base-in or base-out prism power is increased until diplopia or blurred vision is reported. The points at which a break in single vision and a restoration of single vision occur can be measured.

However, diagnosis of the monofixation syndrome requires sensory investigation to identify the presence of a macular scotoma under binocular conditions. Findings on three sensory tests, Worth's four dot test, the four diopter base-out prism test and Bagolini's striated glass test, are summarized in Table 12.1.

Figure 12.1A shows a child with congenital esotropia with an esotropia of greater than 50 prism diopters. Figure 12.1B shows the same patient one week after a bimedial rectus recession who was orthophoric. The patient had the monofixation syndrome and remained within 8 prism diopters of esotropia throughout childhood.

Figure 12.2A shows a patient with a moderate esotropia that is controlled with the appropriate hyperopic correction (accommodative esotropia) (Fig. 12.2B). This patient had the monofixation syndrome with an esotropia less than 8 prism diopters with correction.

Figure 12.3A shows a large nonaccommodative esotropia in a patient with a large macula scar from toxocara (Fig. 12.3B). The patient had strabismus surgery which resulted in the monofixation syndrome and an esotropia of 6 prism diopters with correction.

Table 12.1: Sensory testing in the monofixation syndrome

Worth's Four Dot Test (See Figs 6.2 and 6.3)

- At distant, fixation, the patient sees either 2 or 3 dots. A central scotoma prevents appreciation of the dots imaged in the nonfixating eye
- At near fixation, the patient sees 4 dots. The retinal projection of the dots exceeds the size of the scotoma

Four Diopter Base-Out Prism Test (See Fig. 6.11)

- Absence of movement of one eye is proof of a macular scotoma.
- If the prism is placed in front of the fixating eye, there is initially simultaneous movement of both eyes toward the opposite eye, but no refixation movement of the nonfixating eye occurs.
- If the prism is placed over the nonfixating eye, no movement of either eye occurs.

Bagolini's Striated Glass Test (See Fig. 6.9)

- A gap in the streak of light seen by the nonfixating eye demonstrates scotoma present in the nonfixating eye under binocular conditions

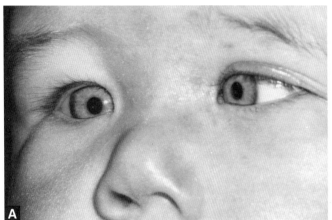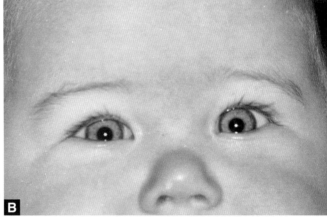

Figs 12.1A and B: Showing a child with congenital esotropia (A) prior to surgery. One week postoperative (B).

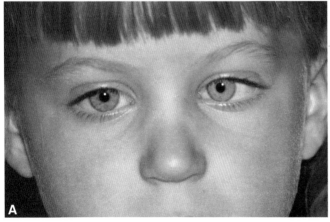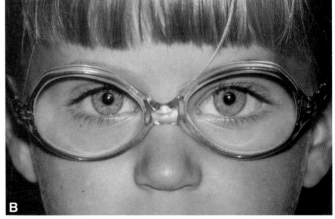

Figs 12.2A and B: Showing a child with accommodative esotropia. Without glasses note the moderate esotropia (A). With glasses note the esotropia was much reduced (B) to within 8 prism diopters of orthophoria.

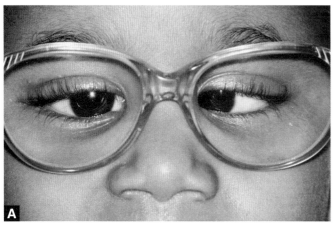 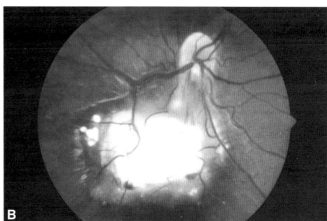

Figs 12.3A and B: Showing a child with a large sensory esotropia (A) from a macular scar (B) following the strabismus surgery, the child had an esotropia of 6 prism diopters.

■ REFERENCE

1. Parks MM. The monofixation syndrome. Trans Am Ophthalmol Soc. 1969;67:609.

■ BIBLIOGRAPHY

1. Mitchell PR, Parks MM. Monofixation syndrome. In: Tasman W, Jaeger EA (Eds). Clinical Ophthalmology. Philadelphia: JB Lippincott Co; 2013.

Syndromes and Special Forms of Strabismus

DUANE'S RETRACTION SYNDROME

Ophthalmic Manifestations

The most characteristic clinical findings in Duane's retraction syndrome (DRS) include a unilateral or bilateral abnormality of horizontal eye movements, retraction of the globe in attempted adduction, and an upward or downward displacement of the globe in adduction. Duane's retraction syndrome occurs more frequently in the left eye than in the right and in females more than males. Bilateral involvement is less frequent than unilateral occurrence. Huber,[1] using electromyography (EMG), has provided a useful classification of DRS into three types.

Type I: Type I DRS is characterized by marked limitation or complete absence of abduction, normal or only slightly restricted adduction, narrowing of the palpebral fissure and retraction of the globe on adduction, and widening of the palpebral fissure on attempted abduction (Fig. 13.1A). Electromyography shows absence of electric activity of the lateral rectus on abduction, but simultaneous firing of the lateral and medial recti on adduction (Fig. 13.1B).

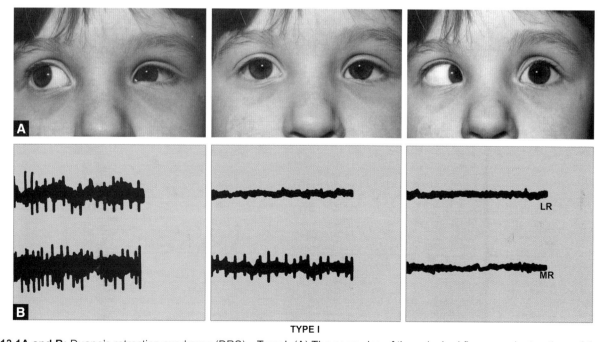

TYPE I

Figs 13.1A and B: Duane's retraction syndrome (DRS)—Type I. (A) The narrowing of the palpebral fissure and retractions of the globe in adduction and the inability to abduct the left eye; (B) The increase contraction of the left medial and lateral rectus in adduction and the absent of contraction in abduction.

Type II: Type II DRS is characterized by limitation or absence of adduction with exotropia of the affected eye, normal or slightly limited abduction, and narrowing of the palpebral fissure and retraction of the affected eye on attempted adduction (Fig. 13.2A). Electromyography reveals contraction of the lateral rectus on both abduction and adduction (Fig. 13.2B).

Type III: Type III DRS is characterized by severe restriction of both abduction and adduction, and retraction of the affected eye and narrowing of the palpebral fissure on attempted adduction. Figure 13.3A shows a patient with Type III DRS of the left eye. Electromyography demonstrates nearly equal contraction of both horizontal recti on both adduction and abduction (Fig. 13.3B).

Figures 13.4A to C show a patient with bilateral Type II DRS. Note the poor adduction of both eyes with mild elevation of the right one in attempted adduction. Figures 13.5A to C show a patient with bilateral Type I DRS with decreased abduction bilaterally.

Type I DRS is the most common, followed in order of frequency by Types II and III. Most patients with Types I and II DRS have straight eyes in the primary position during infancy and childhood. Some children with Type I develop an esodeviation in the primary position and adopt a compensatory head turn toward the side of the involved eye to maintain binocular vision. Children with Type II DRS may develop an exodeviation in the primary position and a face turn away from the involved eye. The upward

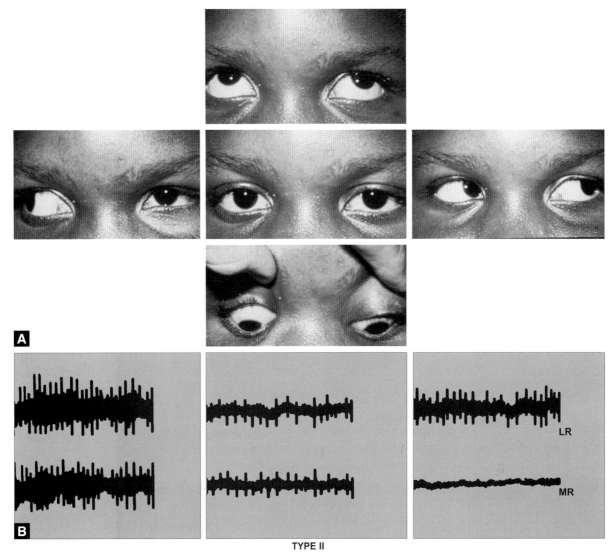

TYPE II

Figs 13.2A and B: Duane's retraction syndrome (DRS)—Type II. (A) The limited adduction of the left eye and normal abduction of the left eye. Note the narrowing of the palpebral fissure on attempted adduction of the left eye; (B) The contraction of the left lateral rectus on both adduction and abduction.

Source: (Fig. 13.2A) Nelson LB, Brown GC, Arentsen JJ. Recognizing patterns of ocular childhood diseases. Thorofare, NJ: Slack, Inc; 1985.

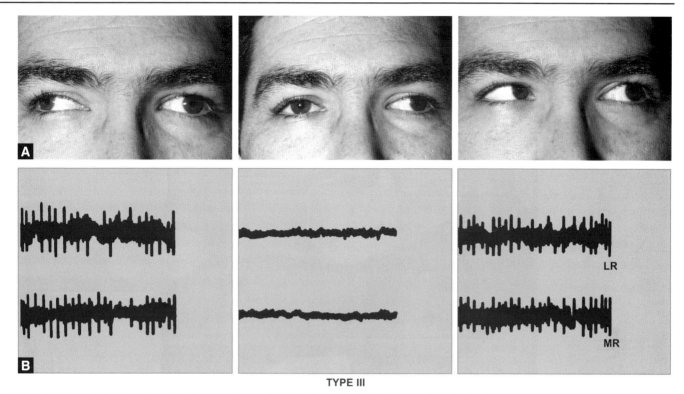

TYPE III

Figs 13.3A and B: Duane's retraction syndrome (DRS)—Type III of the left eye. (A) The inability to adduct or abduct the left eye; (B) Contraction of the left medial and lateral rectus muscles in both adduction and abduction.

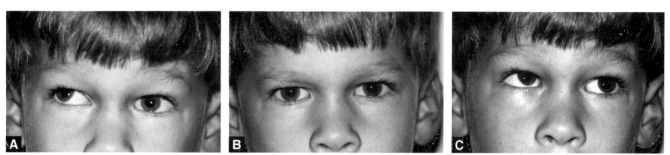

Figs 13.4A to C: Bilateral DRS Type II. Note the limitation of adduction of the left eye (A) and the right eye (C). No strabismus in the primary position (B).

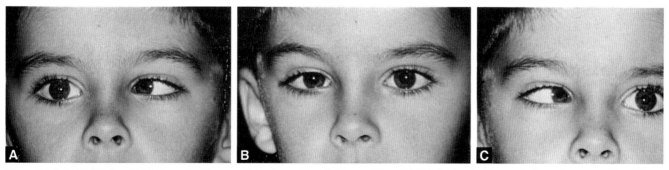

Figs 13.5A to C: Bilateral DRS type I with poor abduction of the right eye (A) and left (C). No strabismus in the primary position (B).

and downward displacements as well as the retraction of the globe on adduction can be as cosmetically distracting as the abnormal head posture.

Figures 13.6A to C show a patient with Type I DRS with significant upward displacement and retraction of the globe on attempted adduction. With more extreme gaze right, the left eye closes almost completely. A patient with Type II DRS with significant downward displacement on attempted adduction is shown in Figures 13.7A to C.

Figures 13.8A to F show a patient with Type III DRS of the left eye. Note the significant retraction of the globe on attempted adduction.

■ BROWN'S SYNDROME

Brown's syndrome is characterized by a congenital or acquired inability to elevate the eye in the adducting position.

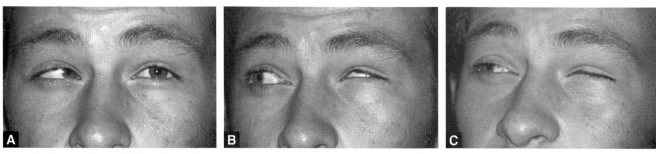

Figs 13.6A to C: Type I DRS with significant leash effect upward of the left eye in adduction.

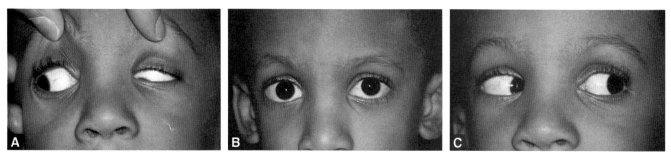

Figs 13.7A to C: Type II DRS with significant downward displacement of the left eye in adduction (A). No strabismus in the primary position (B) and normal abduction of the left eye (C).

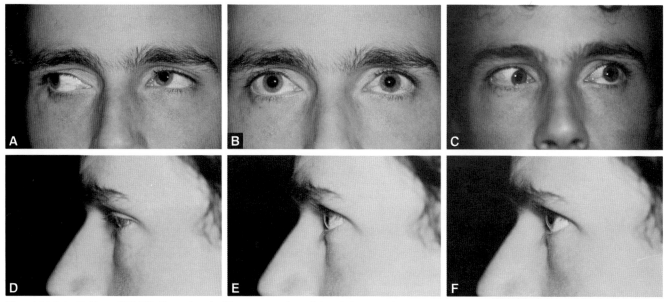

Figs 13.8A to F: Type III DRS. Note the significant retraction of the globe on adduction.

Ophthalmic Manifestations

All features of Brown's syndrome are not necessarily present in any one patient. These features include:

- Limitation of elevation in adduction
- Normal or nearly normal elevation in abduction
- "V" pattern horizontal deviation
- Depression on adduction
- Widening of the palpebral fissure on elevation in adduction
- No overaction of the superior oblique
- Discomfort on attempted elevation in adduction.

A patient with Brown's syndrome of the right eye is shown in Figures 13.9A to I. Note the inability of the right eye to elevate in the adducting position. Elevation of the right eye progressively improves from the straight-up to the abducting position.

A patient with traumatic Brown's syndrome of the right eye is shown in Figures 13.10A to G. This patient had a deep lid laceration in the area of the trochlea, resulting in damage to the right superior oblique tendon. Note the inability to elevate or depress the right eye in the adducting position. Elevation of the right eye improves in both the straight-up and the abducting positions.

■ CYCLIC STRABISMUS

Cyclic strabismus is a rare disorder that is reported to occur in one in 3000–5000 patients with strabismus. Onset usually occurs at 3–4 years of age; most cases with a later age of onset have occurred following surgery or trauma.

Ophthalmic Manifestations

The deviation is, classically, a large-angle esotropia alternating with orthophoria or a small-angle esodeviation on a 48-hour cycle. The duration of the cycle may be as short as 2 weeks or may persist for several years before the deviation becomes constant. Normal binocular vision and good stereoacuity are usually present on the days when the deviation does not occur.

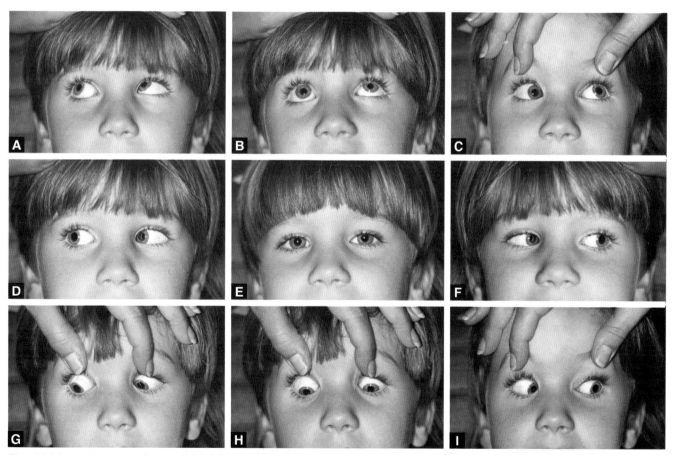

Figs 13.9A to I: Brown syndrome of the right eye. Note the inability to elevate the right eye in adduction (C). Elevation improves in the right eye straight up (B) and abduction (A). No deviation in primary position (E) right (D) or left (F) gaze. Depression normal (H). No superior oblique dysfunction left (G) and right (I) eye.

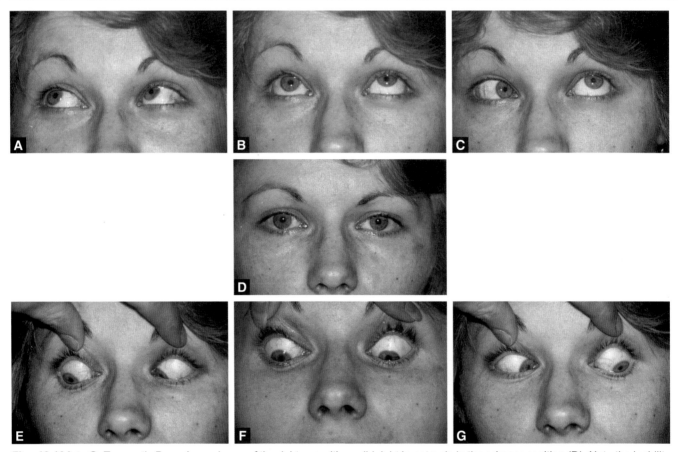

Figs 13.10A to G: Traumatic Brown's syndrome of the right eye with a mild right hypotropia in the primary position (D). Note the inability to elevate (C) or depress (G) the right eye in adduction. Elevation of the right eye improves in the straight up (B) and in the abducting position (A). No abnormality of depression of the right eye in abduction (E) or in direct down-gaze (F).

A 3-year-old girl with cyclic esotropia is shown in Figures 13.11A and B. Note the child was orthophoric (Fig. 13.11A). The following day a large esotropia was noted (Fig. 13.11B).

A child with cyclic esotropia with minimal hyperopic correction on alternate days is shown in Figures 13.12A and B. The patient had strabismus surgery for the amount of esotropia. Postoperatively, the eyes remained orthophoric.

■ MOEBIUS SYNDROME

Moebius syndrome is a rare congenital disturbance, consisting of varying abnormalities of the fifth through the twelfth cranial nerves as well as limb abnormalities.

Ophthalmic Manifestations

Unilateral or bilateral, complete or incomplete facial palsy occurs. Unilateral or bilateral abducent paralysis, either partial or complete, occurs. Esotropia is common.

Figures 13.13A to C show a patient with Moebius syndrome with an esotropia of 45 prism diopters in the primary position. The patient is unable to abduct either eye beyond the midline. This patient also had a seventh nerve palsy, with inability to close the right eye, as shown in Figure 13.14. Note the normal Bell's phenomenon of the right eye.

Systemic Manifestations

Systemic manifestations of Moebius syndrome include:
- Partial atrophy of the tongue, often with inability to protrude the tongue beyond the lips
- Paralysis of the muscles of mastication and of the soft palate (fifth and ninth cranial nerves, respectively)
- Absence or hypoplasia of the pectoral muscles
- Limb anomalies, such as clubfeet, congenital amputations, supernumerary digits, syndactyly and brachydactyly.

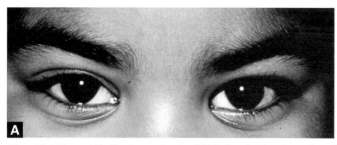
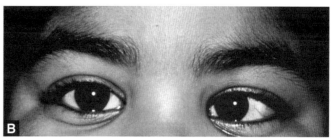

Figs 13.11A and B: Cyclic esotropia. (A) Orthophoria alternating; (B) 24 hours later with esotropia.

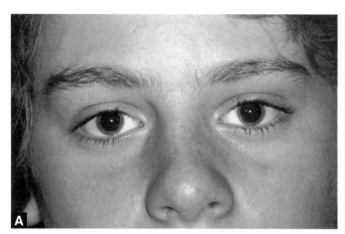
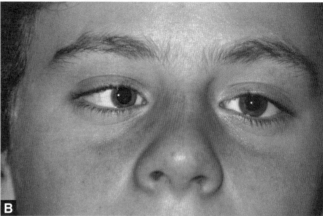

Figs 13.12A and B: Cyclic esotropia with no deviation in primary position. (A) Twenty-four hours later. Note the right esotropia (B).

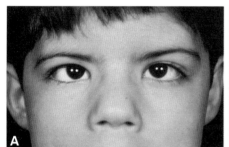
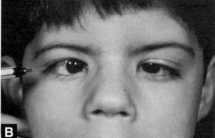
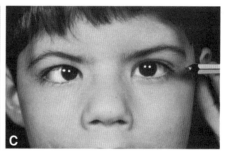

Figs 13.13A to C: Moebius syndrome. Note the esotropia in the primary position (A) and the inability to abduct either eye (B and C).
Source: Nelson LB, Brown GC, Arentsen JJ. Recognizing patterns of ocular childhood diseases. Thorofare, NJ: Slack, Inc; 1985.

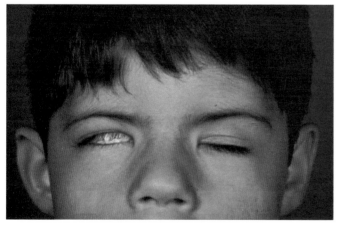

Fig. 13.14: Inability to close the right eye (seventh nerve palsy) in the patient with Moebius syndrome from Figures 13.13A to C.
Source: Nelson LB, Brown GC, Arentsen JJ. Recognizing patterns of ocular childhood diseases. Thorofare, NJ: Slack, Inc; 1985.

Figure 13.15 shows a patient with Moebius syndrome, who has had sucking and feeding problems since infancy. Note the patient's inability to protrude the tongue. Figure 13.16 shows digital abnormalities in a patient with Moebius syndrome.

■ DOUBLE ELEVATOR PALSY

Double elevator palsy is characterized by an inability to elevate the eye in all positions of gaze.

Ophthalmic Manifestations

Ophthalmic manifestations include:
- Limitation of elevation in primary, abducted, and adducted positions, both on versions and ductions
- Hypotropia, frequently present in the primary position
- Pseudoptosis or true ptosis, often present in the primary position
- Chin-up position with fusion in downward gaze or no head position with amblyopia in the hypotropic eye.

A patient with double elevator palsy of the left eye is shown in Figures 13.17A to D. Note the limitation of elevation in all positions of gaze. Figures 13.18A to D show a patient with double elevator palsy of the right eye. Note the apparent right upper eyelid ptosis in the primary position with the left eye fixating. With elevation, the pseudoptosis of the right eyelid disappears. A patient with orbital cellulitis who developed a temporary double elevator palsy of the right eye is shown in Figures 13.19A to G.

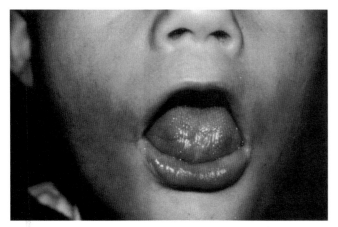

Fig. 13.15: Moebius syndrome with an inability to protrude the tongue.

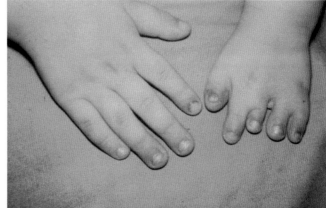

Fig. 13.16: Digital abnormalities in a patient with Moebius syndrome.

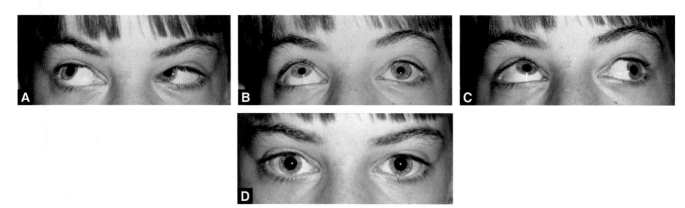

Figs 13.17A to D: Double elevators palsy of the left eye. Note the inability to elevate the left eye in adduction (A), straight up (B), and in abduction (C). No strabismus in the primary position (D).

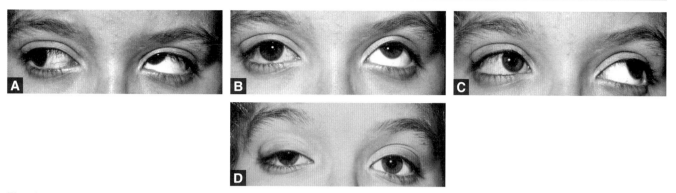

Figs 13.18A to D: Double elevator palsy of the right eye. Pseudoptosis of the right eye with a right hypotropia (D). Ptosis disappears on straight up gaze, (B) Inability to elevate the right eye in abduction (A), straight up (B) in adduction (C).

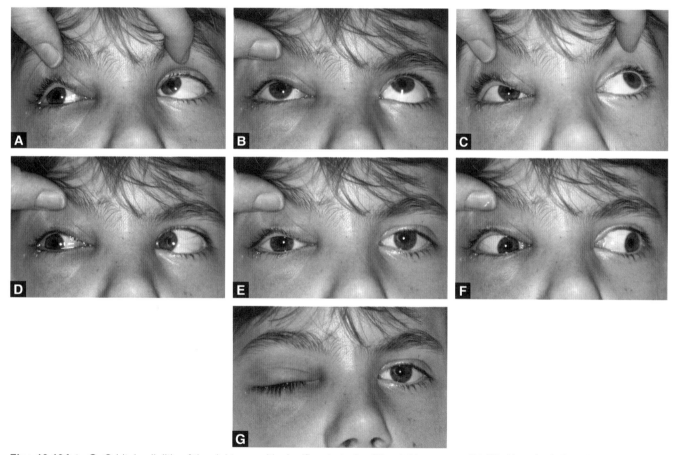

Figs 13.19A to G: Orbital cellulitis of the right eye with significant ptosis of the right upper eyelid (G). Note the induced double elevator palsy of the right eye and the inability to elevate the eye in abduction (A), straight up (B) and adduction (C). No strabismus in right (D) or left gaze (F) or in the primary position (E).

■ THYROID MYOPATHY

Thyroid (endocrine) myopathy is characterized by a limitation of ocular motility, often accompanied by exophthalmos and lid retraction. Figure 13.20 shows extreme exophthalmos and lid retraction in a patient with thyroid disease. This disorder is a common cause of acquired vertical deviation in adults, especially females, and a rare cause of acquired vertical deviation in children.

Ophthalmic Manifestations

Esotropia, hypotropia, or a combination of both occurs. The most commonly affected extraocular muscle is the inferior rectus followed by the medial rectus. Figure 13.21 shows a woman with thyroid myopathy with inferior rectus involvement and a large hypotropia in primary position. Usually, there is a positive forced duction test because of pathologic changes in the extraocular muscles.

Werner classified the eye and orbital findings in thyroid myopathy and summarized these, using the acronym — "NO SPECS" (Box 13.1).[2]

Figure 13.22 shows exophthalmos, lid retraction and right hypotropia in a patient with hyperthyroidism. Figure 13.23 shows a computed tomography (CT) scan that demonstrates the thickened horizontal rectus muscles, especially the medial recti, in a patient with hyperthyroidism.

■ BLOWOUT FRACTURES

Blowout fractures are produced when a blunt object, such as a baseball or a fist, strikes the orbital rim and causes a sudden increase in intraorbital pressure. The force applied

Box 13.1: Ocular and orbital findings in thyroid disease
N—No signs
O—Only signs (upper lid retraction and stare, with or without lid lag and proptosis)
S—Soft tissue involvement (signs and symptoms)
P—Proptosis
E—Extraocular muscle involvement
C—Corneal involvement
S—Sight loss (optic nerve involvement)

Source: Werner SC. Classification of the eye changes of Graves' disease. J Clin Endocrinol Metab. 1969;29:782.

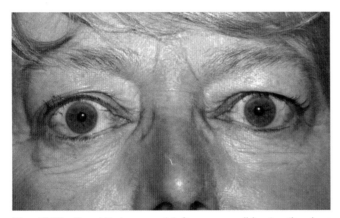

Fig. 13.20: Exophthalmos and left upper eyelid retraction in a patient with thyroid myopathy.
Courtesy: Jacqueline Carrasco MD.

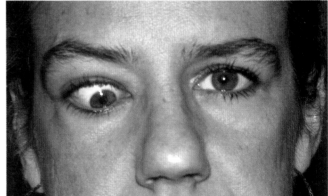

Fig. 13.21: Large hypotropia with thyroid myopathy.
Courtesy: Jacqueline Carrasco MD.

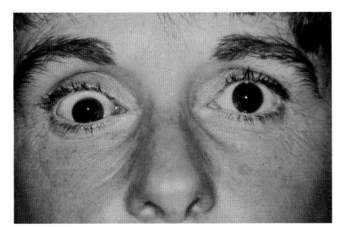

Fig. 13.22: Large right hypotropia and left upper eyelid retraction in a patient with thyroid myopathy.
Courtesy: Jacqueline Carrasco MD.

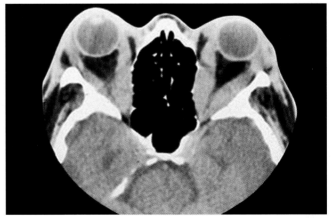

Fig. 13.23: CT scan of a patient with thyroid myopathy. Note the thickened horizontal muscles: especially both medial rectus muscles and right lateral rectus muscle.
Courtesy: Mary Stefanyszyn MD.

to the orbit is transferred to the bony orbital walls. The medial wall (lamina papyracea) and the orbital floor (roof of the maxillary antrum) are the weakest bones of the orbit and are damaged most frequently.

Blunt trauma applied to the anterior orbit results in a blowout fracture with incarceration of the inferior rectus and orbital fat (Fig. 13.24). This helps explain the restriction of vertical motility and a positive forced duction test. Figure 13.25 shows a CT scan demonstrating a blowout fracture of the left orbit.

Figures 13.26A to E show a patient with entrapment of the left inferior rectus that prevented normal elevation of the left eye in all positions. There is a large hypotropia in primary gaze. A contusion injury to the inferior rectus also prevents full depression of the left eye.

■ MARCUS GUNN'S SYNDROME

Marcus Gunn's (jaw-winking) syndrome consists of blepharoptosis in which there is retraction of the affected eyelid in conjunction with stimulation of the ipsilateral

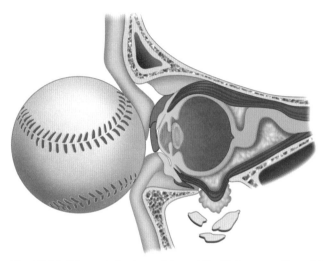

Fig. 13.24: Blowout fracture of the orbit with incarceration of the inferior rectus muscle.
Artist: Karen Albert.
Source: Nelson LB. Pediatric Ophthalmology. Philadelphia: WB Saunders Co; 1984.

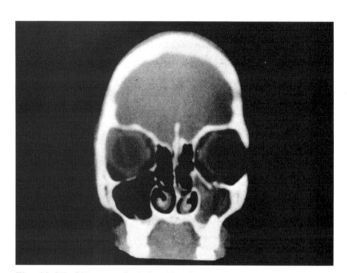

Fig. 13.25: CT scan of a left orbital fracture.
Courtesy: Mary Stefanyszyn MD.

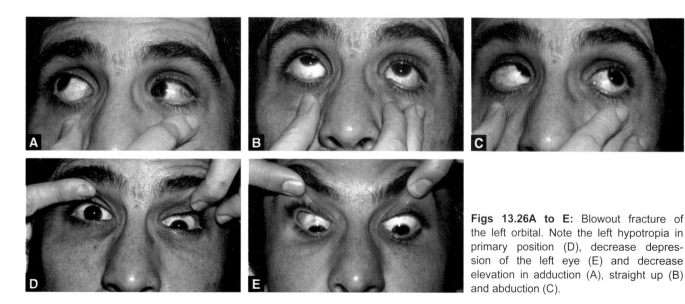

Figs 13.26A to E: Blowout fracture of the left orbital. Note the left hypotropia in primary position (D), decrease depression of the left eye (E) and decrease elevation in adduction (A), straight up (B) and abduction (C).

pterygoid muscle. It is caused by an abnormal interconnection between the third and fifth cranial nerves.

Ophthalmic Manifestations

Ophthalmic manifestations include:
- Occurrence in 2–13% of patients with ptosis
- Unilateralism, commonly
- Ptosis with retraction of the affected eyelid as a result of opening the mouth, chewing, sucking, or movement of the jaw toward the contralateral side
- Associated ocular abnormalities, such as amblyopia, double elevator palsy and superior rectus palsy.

Figures 13.27A to F show a patient with jaw-winking syndrome of the right upper eyelid. Note that when the jaw moves to the left, the right upper eyelid elevates. Note that with progressive jaw movement to the left, the right upper eyelid elevates more.

■ GENERALIZED FIBROSIS SYNDROME

Generalized fibrosis syndrome is characterized by replacement of normal muscle tissue by fibrous tissue in varying degrees. The various clinical presentations depend on the number of muscles affected, the degree of fibrosis, and whether the involvement is unilateral or bilateral.

Ophthalmic Manifestations

Ophthalmic manifestations include:
- Fibrosis of the extraocular muscles and Tenon's capsule
- Inelasticity and fragility of the conjunctiva
- Absence of elevation or depression of the eyes
- Little or no horizontal movement
- Blepharoptosis or pseudoptosis with chin elevation
- Exotropia or esotropia, frequently
- Amblyopia, commonly. When there are significant refractive errors, amblyopia may be partly due to the

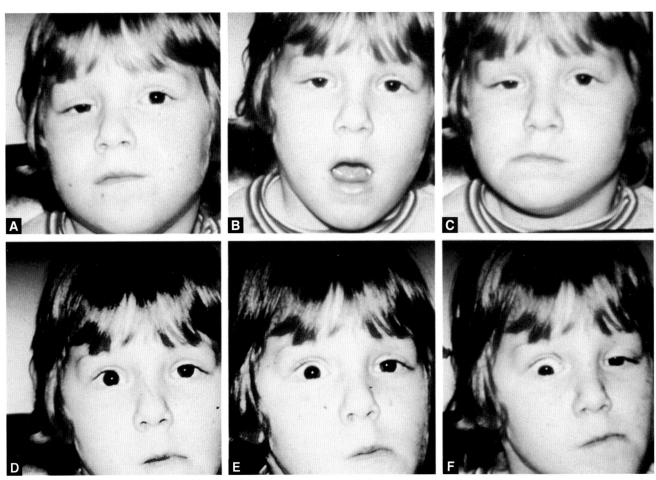

Figs 13.27A to F: Marcus Gunn's syndrome of the right eye (A) Opening of the mouth, the right eyelid elevates minimally (B) when the jaw moves to the right, the ptosis of the right upper eyelid is unchanged (C). When the jaw moves to the left (D to F), the right upper eyelid elevates.
Source: Harley RD. Disorders of the lids. Pediatr Clin North Am. 1983;30:114.

difficulty of wearing an optical correction device, with the head in an extended chin-up position.

A child with generalized fibrosis syndrome is shown in Figures 13.28A to D. Note the chin-up position, which is decreased on attempted upward gaze, and accentuated on attempted downward gaze.

Severe generalized fibrosis syndrome is shown in Figures 13.29A to D. The child maintains a chin-up position to fixate (Figs 13.29A and B).

Figures 13.29B to D show primary position with the left eye fixating and a large exotropia. Left and right gaze shows minimal lateral movement of the eyes.

■ CHRONIC PROGRESSIVE EXTERNAL OPHTHALMOPLEGIA

Chronic progressive external ophthalmoplegia (CPEO) is characterized by insidiously progressive, symmetric immobility of the eyes, which do not move even with oculocephalic or caloric stimulation.

Ophthalmic Manifestations

Ophthalmoplegia is slowly progressive and symmetric and is usually associated with ptosis and orbicularis weakness. Retinal pigmentary degeneration occurs as well.

Systemic Manifestations

Systemic manifestations of CPEO include cardiac conduction defects, elevated cerebrospinal fluid protein and spongiform encephalopathy, including the brainstem.

A patient with CPEO with complete ptosis of the right eye is shown in Figure 13.30. There is an almost complete absence of eye movements in all fields of gaze.

Figures 13.31A to C show the same patient with CPEO in Figure 13.30 with a large exotropia in primary position with little horizontal movement of the eyes. Figures 13.32A to E show a patient with CPEO with bilateral severe ptosis and almost no eye movements.

Figure 13.33 shows pigment clumping in the retina of a patient with CPEO.

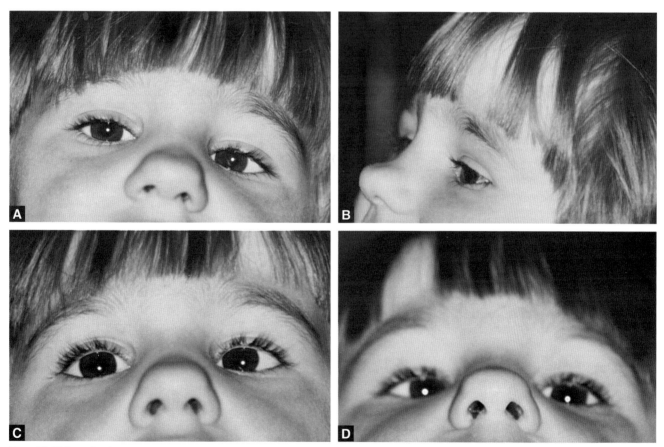

Figs 13.28A to D: Generalized fibrosis syndrome. Large chin-up position with inability to move either eye in any position. Chin-up position in primary position (A and B). On attempted up-gaze, mild decrease in the chin-up position (C). On attempted down-gaze, increase in chin-up position (D).

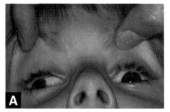
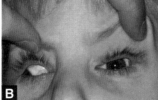
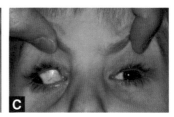
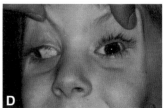

Figs 13.29A to D: Generalized fibrosis syndrome chin-up position (A) in order to fixate. With head in the straight-ahead position, the right eye remains in the exotropic position (D). Minimal movement of the eyes in right gaze (B) or left gaze (C).

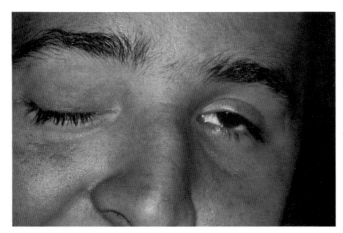

Fig. 13.30: CPEO with complete closure of the right eye.

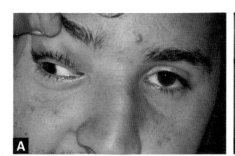
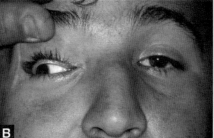
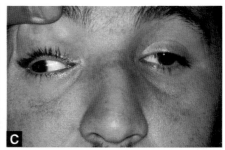

Figs 13.31A to C: Patient with CPEO from Figure 13.30 with almost no eye movements in any position of gaze (A to C). Minimal movement of the eyes in right gaze (A). Large exotropia in primary position (B). Almost no movement in left gaze (C).

PARINAUD'S SYNDROME

This dorsal midbrain syndrome is characterized by a supra-nuclear vertical gaze paresis with nuclear oculomotor pare-ses and pupillomotor abnormalities. Parinaud's syndrome is due to midbrain tegmentum, periaqueductal and poste-rior commissure lesions. In children, Parinaud's syndrome is especially seen with pinealoma and aqueductal stenosis.

Ophthalmic Manifestations

- Upward gaze is reduced, with preservation of downward gaze. A doll's head maneuver or Bell's phenomenon does elevate the eyes

- Attempts at upward gaze produce variable degrees of retraction-convergence nystagmus
- Palpebral fissure widening occurs on attempted upward gaze (Collier's sign)
- Dissociation of the light near response occurs; pupils are mid-dilated and fixated to light but react normally to accommodative effort.

A patient with Parinaud's syndrome, with defective upward gaze but normal downward gaze and horizontal movement, is shown in Figures 13.34A to E. Note the convergence on attempted upward gaze. A doll's head maneuver demonstrates normal vertical movements in this patient (Figs 13.35A and B).

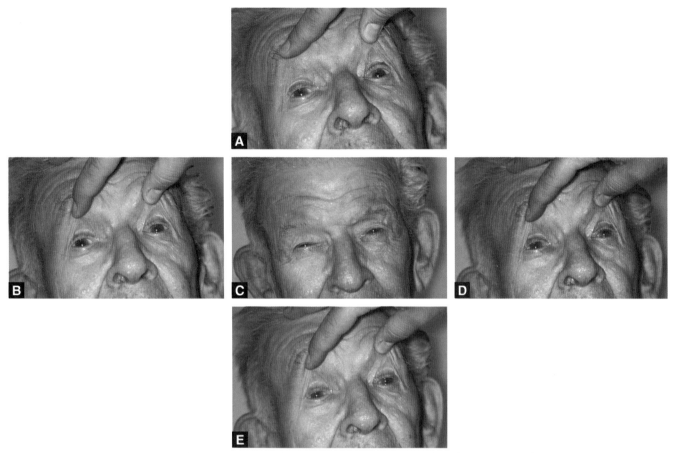

Figs 13.32A to E: Patient with CPEO with severe ptosis and minimal eye movement in all fields of gaze. Exotropia in primary position (A). No movement in right (B) or left gaze (D). Severe ptosis in primary position (C). No depression ability (E).

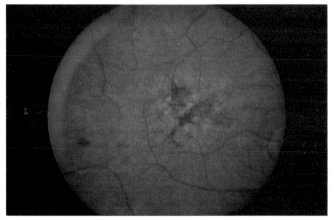

Fig. 13.33: Pigment clumping in the retina in a patient with CPEO.

INTERNUCLEAR OPHTHALMOPLEGIA

Internuclear ophthalmoplegia (INO) is characterized by impaired adduction on attempted contralateral gaze, with horizontal nystagmus in the abducting eye. Vertical nystagmus on attempted upward gaze is often concomitant. Adduction on convergence is frequently preserved. Internuclear ophthalmoplegia is believed to be caused by a lesion in the medial longitudinal fasciculus.

Figures 13.36A to I show unilateral INO in a patient 2 days after an automobile accident. Note the inability of the right eye to adduct fully on left gaze. Convergence, however, is normal (Fig. 13.37).

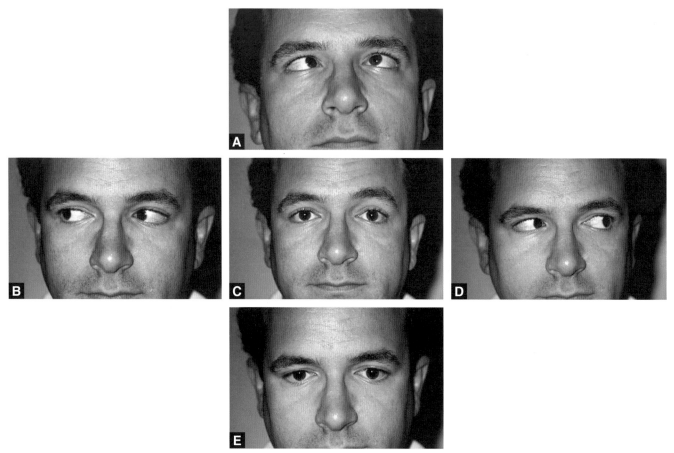

Figs 13.34A to E: Parinaud's syndrome in a patient with inability to elevate (A) with normal horizontal movement. Note convergence on attempted up-gaze (A). No abnormality in right (B) or left (D) gaze. Orthophoria in primary position (C). Down-gaze is normal (E).

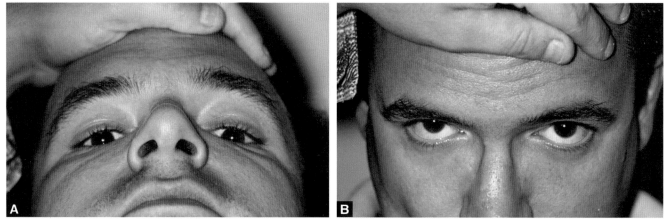

Figs 13.35A and B: Same patient in Figures 13.34A to E with Parinaud's syndrome with no vertical movement had normal depression (A) and elevation (B) with Doll's head maneuver.

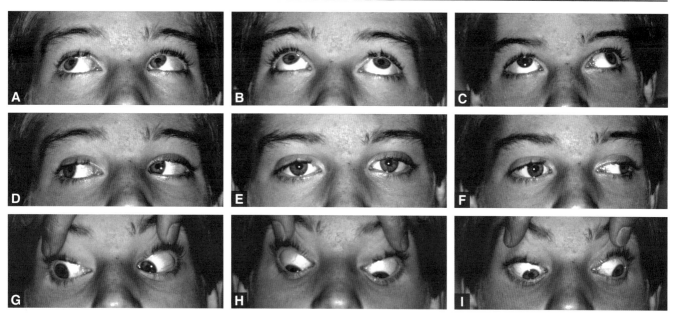

Figs 13.36A to I: Right INO. Note the inability to adduct the right eye completely (A to F). Normal ability to elevate and depress in right gaze (A and G) and left gaze (C and I) elevation (B) and depression (H) are normal. Adduction of the left eye is normal (D). No strabismus in primary position (E).
Source: Catalano RA, Sax RD, Krohel GB. Unilateral internuclear ophthalmoplegia after head trauma. Am J Ophthalmol. 1986;101:491.

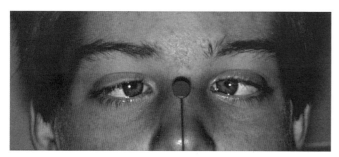

Fig. 13.37: Same patient with INO from Figures 13.36 A to I with normal convergence.
Source: Catalano RA, Sax RD, Krohel GB. Unilateral internuclear ophthalmoplegia after head trauma. Am J Ophthalmol. 1986;101:491. (Published with permission from The American Journal of Ophthalmology).

■ REFERENCES

1. Huber A. Electrophysiology of the retraction syndrome. Br J Ophthalmol. 1974;58:293.
2. Werner SC. Classification of the eye changes of Graves' disease. J Clin Endocrinol Metab. 1969;29:782.

■ BIBLIOGRAPHY

1. Brown HW. True and simulated superior oblique tendon sheath syndromes. Doc Ophthalmol. 1973;34:123.
2. Friendly DS, Manson RA, Albert DG. Cyclic strabismus: a case study . Doc Ophthalmol. 1973;34:189.
3. Glaser JS. Infranuclear disorders of eye movement. In: Tasman W, Jaeger EA (Eds). Clinical Ophthalmology. Philadelphia: JB Lippincott Co; 2013.
4. Harley RD, Rodrigues MM, Crawford JS. Congenital fibrosis of the extraocular muscles. Trans Am Ohthalmol Soc. 1978; 76:197.
5. Henderson JH. The congenital facial diplegia syndrome: clinical features, pathology, and aetiology: a review of sixty-one cases. Brain. 1939;62:381.
6. Hotchkiss MG, Miller NR, Clark AW, et al. Bilateral Duane's retraction syndrome: a clinical-pathologic case report. Arch Ophthalmol. 1980;98:870.
7. Huber A. Electrophysiology of the retraction syndrome. Br J Ophthalmol. 1974;9:293.
8. Isenberg S, Urist MJ. Clinical observations in 101 consecutive patients with Duane's retraction syndrome. Am J Ophthalmol. 1977;84:419.
9. Kearns TP. External ophthalmoplegia, pigmentary degeneration of the retina and cardiomyopathy: a newly recognized syndrome. Trans Am Ophthalmol Soc. 1965;65:559.
10. Miller NR, Kiel SM, Green WR, et al. Unilateral Duane's retraction syndrome (type 1). Arch Ophthalmol. 1982;100:2468.
11. Mitchell PR, Parks MM. Ophthalmologic syndromes and trauma. In: Tasman W, Jaeger EA (Eds). Clinical Ophthalmology. Philadelphia: JB Lippincott Co; 2013.
12. Parks MM, Eustis HS. Simultaneous superior oblique tenotomy and inferior oblique recession in Brown's syndrome. Ophthalmol. 1987;94:1043.
13. Pratt SG, Beyer CK, Johnson CC. The Marcus Gunn phenomenon: a review of 71 cases. Ophthalmol. 1984;90:27.
14. Scott WE, Jackson OB. Double elevator palsy: the significance of inferior rectus restriction. Am Orthoptic J. 1977;27:5.
15. Sergott RC, Glaser JS. Graves' ophthalmopathy: a clinical and immunologic review. Surv Ophthalmol. 1981;26:1.
16. von Noorden GK, Campos EC. Binocular Vision and Ocular Motility, 6th edition. St. Louis, Mo: CV Mosby; 2002.

Index

Page numbers followed by *f* refer to figure and *t* refer to table.